Intersex
in the Age of
Ethics

Ethics in Clinical Medicine Series

Intersex in the Age of Ethics

Edited by

Alice Domurat Dreger

University Publishing Group
Hagerstown, Maryland

University Publishing Group, Inc.
Hagerstown, Maryland 21740
1-800-654-8188

ISBN (cloth): 1-55572-125-7
ISBN (paper): 1-55572-100-1

Chapters 1 through 4, 12, 15 through 17, and 21 first appeared in *The Journal of
Clinical Ethics* 9, no. 4 (Winter 1998); © 1998 by *The Journal of Clinical Ethics;*
used with permission.
Earlier versions of the following chapters were published in *Chrysalis: The Journal of Transgressive Gender Identities* 2, no. 5 (Fall 1997/Winter 1998): chapter 5
© 1998 by Martha Coventry; chapter 6 © 1998 by Howard Devore; chapter 8 ©
1998 by D. Cameron; chapter 10 © 1998 by Tamara Alexander; chapter 13 ©
1998 by Angela Moreno; chapter 14 © 1998 by Kiira Triea; chapter 20 © 1998
by Sven Nicholson; used with the permission of the individual authors.
Chapter 18 © 1998 by Helena Harmon-Smith; used with permission.
An earlier version of chapter 19 was published as "Physically Screwed by Cultural Myth: The Story of a Buffalo Children's Hospital Survivor," in *Hermaphrodites with Attitude* (Fall-Winter 1995-1996): 10-11; © 1996 by ISNA; used with
permission.

Photo credits: pp. 7, 8—figures 1-1 and 1-2 originally appeared in T. Tuffier and
A. Lapointe, "L'Hermaphrodisme: Ses variétés et ses conséquences pour la pratique médicale (d'après un cas personnel)," *Revue de gynécologie et de chirurgie
abdominale* 17 (1911): 209-68; p. 156—(A) is reprinted from K. Newman, J.
Randolph, and K. Anderson, "The Surgical Management of Infants and Children with Ambiguous Genitalia: Lessons Learned from 25 Years," *Annals of
Surgery* 215, no. 6 (1992): 644-53, at 647, fig. 6, © 1992 by Lippincott Williams
& Wilkins, used with permission; (B), (C), and (D) © 1998 by ISNA, used with
permission.

This volume is dedicated to Cheryl Chase
and to those who have had the courage
to speak with her and listen to her.

Contents

Part 3: Changing Perspectives of the Clinic

Part 4: What to Do Now

Acknowledgments

I am grateful to the staff of University Publishing Group and *The Journal of Clinical Ethics* for their invaluable assistance in producing this volume. Edmund Howe suggested and encouraged the original collection. Norman Quist has been tremendously supportive throughout the long and convoluted process of publishing a book with 22 different authors and a whole lot of photos. (He said "yes" to everything, even orange.) April McNamee and Heather Green held up beautifully under the pressure of many a bizarre e-mail. And Leslie LeBlanc has truly earned the title of "Glenda, the Good Witch of Publishing." Without Leslie, this volume would not exist, and I would not be smiling while wrapping up the final bits.

Chapters 1 through 4, 12, 15 through 17, and 21 of this book originally appeared in a Special Issue on Intersexuality in *The Journal of Clinical Ethics*, for which I was the special editor. Some of these chapters have been slightly updated and revised.

Earlier versions of chapters 5, 6, 8, 10, 13, 14, and 20 were collected and edited by Martha Coventry and Cheryl Chase for a Special Issue on Intersexuality of *Chrysalis: The Journal of Transgressive Gender Identities*. I am grateful to Martha Coventry and Cheryl Chase for their work on these essays, and to Dallas Denny, Publisher and Editor in Chief of *Chrysalis*.

Chapter 18 originally appeared on the website of the Hermaphrodite Education and Listening Post (HELP) < http://www.help@jaxnet .com >.

An earlier version of chapter 19 was published as "Physically Screwed by Cultural Myth: The Story of a Buffalo Children's Hospital Survivor," in the journal *Hermaphrodites with Attitude*.

I would also like to acknowledge the kind assistance of the Wangensteen Historical Library at the University of Minnesota in Minneapolis for providing prints for figures 1-1 and 1-2.

Financial and moral support for this work has been provided by the Lyman Briggs School and the College of Natural Science of Michigan

State University. I am also grateful for the support of the staff and faculty of the Center for Ethics and Humanities in the Life Sciences at Michigan State University, especially Libby Bogdan-Lovis and Howard Brody. The Enhancement Technologies and Human Identity Working Group has helped me with this project in indirect but critical ways; for their companionship, feedback, and encouragement I am very thankful (and I promise Tod Chambers I will go free the Irish Giant as soon as I finish typing this).

The authors of this volume have been wonderfully dependable and enthusiastic. I am grateful to them for sharing their experiences, talents, and visions.

Finally, I am tremendously indebted to two people, Aron Sousa, my mate, and Cheryl Chase, who as a tag team kept me going by pushing and pulling, helping with ideas, proofreading, and correspondence. Now that we're done with this, perhaps the two of you can try to explain land tides to me again.

PART 1

Intersex as a
Social Phenomenon

Introduction to Part 1

People who treat, study, and live with intersex agree that intersexed genitals are troubling not because intersexed genitals are diseased, but because they look different. A cultural system that depends on two and only two gender categories, which in turn depend on two and only two sex categories, reacts to intersex—the blurring of sex distinctions—with revulsion, panic, and sometimes "normalizing" medicine.

In part 1 of this volume, the opening essay by Alice Domurat Dreger lays out a skeletal history of the biomedical treatment of intersex, and traces the three most recent eras of this treatment: the Age of Gonads, in which the Victorians hoped to "solve" blurry sex by relying on gonadal tissue to tell them who was male and who female; the Age of Surgery, in which doctors thought they could make any body conform to male and female gender roles if only they could surgically and hormonally make the body look more male or female; and the emerging Age of Consent, in which the chief concern is no longer to medically sort everyone into male and female body types, but in which the chief concern is rather to value the autonomy of the intersexed person.

In the first of many essays by intersexuals in this volume, Sherri Groveman compares the social aspects of being intersexed with the social aspects of being Jewish. Using the stories of many women like her with androgen insensitivity syndrome (AIS), Groveman demonstrates that, however well intentioned, the Age of Surgery system of treatment involves the violation of basic ethical principles, most importantly the principle of truth-telling.

Robert Crouch expands on Groveman's analysis, using the tools of anthropologists in an effort to understand why the reaction to intersex has been so strong and so troubled. Sociologist Sharon Preves rounds out the critiques offered by Crouch and Groveman by summarizing her in-depth interviews with 41 adults born intersexed. Preves shows that the treatment does not always achieve the desired effect of happiness for patients. She also traces the process by which increasing numbers of intersexuals are beginning to "come out" and construct an intersex rights movement.

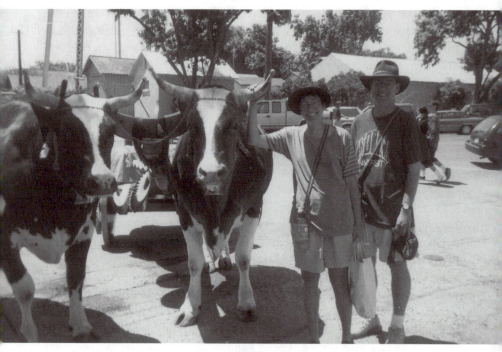

Alice Domurat Dreger and Aron Sousa

1

A History of Intersex: From the Age of Gonads to the Age of Consent

Alice Domurat Dreger

This marks the first time an entire volume has been dedicated to the exploration of the ethics of intersex treatment. It could not be more timely; professional conferences, gender clinics, and the popular media are abuzz with the controversy over how medicine and society should handle intersex and intersexuals. The volume will provide some much-needed perspective.

The chapters that follow explain the phenomena known collectively as intersexuality in some depth. For the uninitiated, I will simply note here that "hermaphroditism" and "intersex" are blanket terms used to denote a variety of congenital conditions in which a person has neither the standard male nor the standard female anatomy. Of course, what counts as "standard" male or female is open to interpretation. How big does a "clitoris" have to be before it is "non-standard"—and is size all you should count? Should facial hair be considered "standard" in men and not in women and children, even though some men have little facial hair and some women much? Should our "standards" of sex be based on hidden parts like gonads or chromosomes even though most of us don't know with certainty the nature of our gonads and chromosomes?

Questions such as these become more numerous and more difficult as one investigates the myriad of human sex variations. In fact, because of ever-more discoveries of sexual variation and ever-more developments in sexual politics, medical and lay definitions of "male" and "female" have changed repeatedly and continue to change. These definitional shifts have been driven by technological and theoretical advances in biomedical fields (for example, genetics), but they have also been driven by anxious responses to hermaphroditism. As I've learned from nearly nine years of study, intersexuality messes up just about every rule you have been led to believe about sex and gender. Anxiety ensues, and often in reaction to this anxiety, non-intersexuals have demanded order out of intersexuals.

THE AGE OF GONADS

Consider what happened in France and Britain in the late 19th century. At that time, medical doctors were already feeling rather worried about the instability of political-sexual identities. The recently named "homosexual" was showing up in alarming numbers, and a vocal minority of women agitated for equal rights under the law, in the professions, and in the universities. During this already anxious time, doctors started to discover an astonishing number of physically hermaphroditic subjects. As I argue in *Hermaphrodites and the Medical Invention of Sex*,[1] this was due in part to the rise of gynecology and the fact that more people were seeing doctors. But anxiety about sex roles probably also contributed to the rapid rise in medical reports of hermaphrodites by making physicians sensitive to their patients' sexual identities, anatomies, and practices.

In an effort to forestall physical sexual confusion (hermaphroditism) lest it amplify social sexual confusion, biomedical experts in the late 19th century groped around looking for stable and non-overlapping definitions of "male," "female," and "true hermaphrodite." Only if non-overlapping categories could be found would the two-sex social system truly be safe. Apparent salvation came in the form of what I call the Gonadal Definition of Sex.

In 1896, led by two British experts, George F. Blacker (1865-1948) and T.W.P. Lawrence (1858-1936), American and European medical men rallied around the idea that the anatomical nature of the gonads (as ovarian or testicular) alone should determine a subject's "true sex," no matter how confusing or mixed her or his other parts. Henceforth, no matter how manly a patient looked, even if he had a full-sized penis, no vagina, a full beard, and a reputation for bedding down (and satisfying) young maidens, if he had ovaries, he would be labeled a female—in this

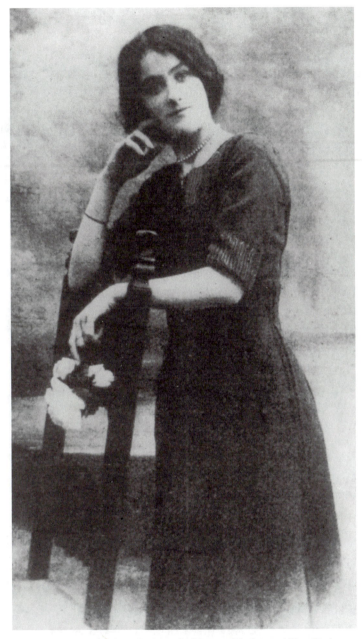

Figure 1-1. Photograph of L.S., a Parisian fashion model, deemed "frankly homosexual" by French medical experts in 1911 because she sexually desired men and not women. L.S. had testicles, and so was labeled a "male pseudo-hermaphrodite."

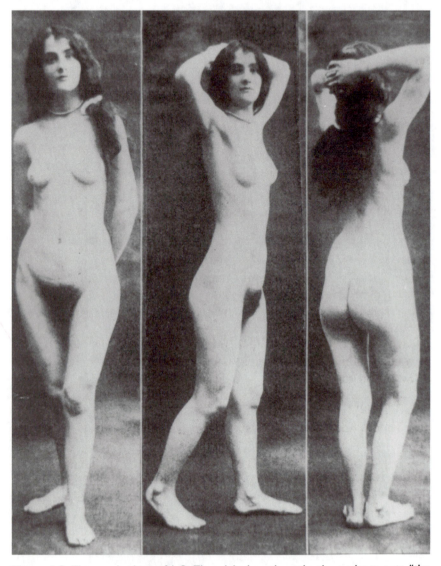

Figure 1-2. Three nude shots of L.S. The original caption asks the reader to note "the virilism" of the lower limbs, "in particular the feet."

case a "female pseudo-hermaphrodite." No matter how womanly a patient looked, no matter if she had a vagina, fine and rounded breasts, a smooth face, and a husband she loved, if she had testes, she would be labeled a male—in this case a "male pseudo-hermaphrodite" (for an example of a "male pseudo-hermaphrodite," see figures 1.1 and 1.2).[2]

So strong was doctors' belief in the Gonadal Definition of Sex and the primacy of the gonads that in Britain the "problem" of "women" with testes was sometimes "solved" by removing the testes from these women, and in France by imploring these patients to stop their "homosexual" alliances with men.[3] (As you might guess, incredulous hermaphroditic patients sometimes thought their doctors daft or cruel.) Commenting on the case of L.S. (shown in figures 1.1 and 1.2), a testes-laden woman labeled by her doctors "frankly homosexual" because she passionately loved only men, a pair of French experts observed, "The possession of a [single] sex [as male or female] is a necessity of our social order, for hermaphrodites as well as for normal subjects."[4] And so nearly everyone would be labeled male or female, even if pseudo (falsely) hermaphroditic.

During this Age of Gonads, the only "true hermaphrodite" was that subject whose gonads—upon *microscopic* verification by *teams* of experts—were confirmed to contain both ovarian and testicular tissue. Non-emergency exploratory surgeries were quite rare, and biopsies basically unheard of; and so, conveniently, the only true hermaphrodite was a dead hermaphrodite, or at least a castrated (and therefore non?) hermaphrodite. With this intellectual set-up, most sexually challenging patients could be labeled "truly" male or female, and only in the most unlikely and extraordinarily of cases would a patient be labeled "truly hermaphroditic."

Surely this Gonadal Definition came about in 1896 in part because of recent discoveries in endocrinological and embryological research. The gonads looked to be pretty important physiologically and developmentally, and certainly they are. But allegiance to science alone cannot explain the fierce adherence to the Gonadal Definition. For doctors did not care if the ovarian or testicular tissue in any given patient *functioned*, nor did they ever give up on believing that sex signs showed up all over the body—on the face, the chest, in the tastes, desires, and behaviors, even (in some professional minds) in the color of the fingernails and the bend of the knee. Doctors liked the Gonadal Definition because it kept almost every living body to only one "true" sex, male or female.[5]

Again, note that *only* claims of *true* hermaphroditism required microscopes and teams of experts. The identity of "male" or "female" (even if "pseudo-hermaphroditic") was seen as largely unproblematic; labeling patients truly male or female kept the sexes down to the safe number of two, and so it was pretty easy for a doctor to label a patient "male" or "female" without his colleagues giving him grief. But try to label a patient truly hermaphroditic, and the wrath of the high-powered and numerous defenders of the Gonadal Definition would rain down. One living body, one sex. That was the rule. Sex stabilized. Problem solved.

Well, not quite. Advancing technologies soon made it possible to discover and verify living true hermaphrodites via tissue-sparing biopsies, and doctors started to question what it would mean for social order to label a living person a "true hermaphrodite" or an astoundingly womanly patient (like L.S.) "male" just because she had testes. Thanks to the new diagnostic technologies, the old Gonadal Definition of Sex was failing.

By 1915, one physician harkened the end of the Age of Gonads by raising the question of whether doctors shouldn't abandon the Gonadal Definition. William Blair Bell (1871-1939), then staff surgeon to the Royal Infirmary at Liverpool, considered the latest findings of endocrinology and the trouble caused by the new diagnostic technologies, and wrote, "Since it is now possible to demonstrate the fact that the psychical and physical attributes of sex are not necessarily dependent on the gonads, I think that each case should be considered as a whole; that is to say, the sex should be determined by the obvious predominance of characteristics, especially the secondary, and not by the non-functional sex-glands alone, for this is neither scientific nor just."[6]

In spite of his revolutionary prescription for sex diagnosis, one that moved overtly and consciously away from the Gonadal Definition, Blair Bell's position was conservative in two fundamental ways. First, Blair Bell was, like his predecessors, motivated in theory and practice by an interest in maintaining clear, medically sanctioned divisions between the two sexes in each individual case and in society as a whole. Indeed, this was largely the reason Blair Bell suggested the abandonment of the gonad-as-exclusive-marker rule. It didn't work anymore. Like his colleagues, Blair Bell wanted to quiet sex anomalies, not accentuate them as the Gonadal Definition now threatened to do.

Second, Blair Bell maintained the idea that every body did indeed have a *single true sex*, even if "neither the sex-gland nor the genital ducts necessarily influence or give any indication of the true sex of the individual, as shown by the secondary characteristics."[7] Blair Bell recommended that medical doctors not only diagnose a single sex for anomalous bodies, but that they then *help it along*, by eliminating any sexually "anomalous" characteristics and accenting those that matched the so-diagnosed sex. Blair Bell concluded, "our opinion of the gender [of a given patient] should be adapted to the peculiar circumstances and to our modern knowledge of the complexity of sex, and surgical procedures should in these special cases be carried out to establish more completely the obvious sex of the individual."[8]

So, "true sex" would, perhaps, no longer be dictated exclusively by the anatomical nature of the gonads, but only two true sexes would still exist, with a limit of one to each body, and the medical expert would still be the interpreter—and now, when necessary and possible, the amplifier—of true sex.

TO THE AGE OF SURGERY

This—the assignment to and the surgical construction of a single, believable sex for each ambiguous body—was indeed the wave of the future. Blair Bell's work sounded the end of the Age of Gonads, and it harkened in a successor era that we could call the Age of Surgery. In this period—still going on today—each body would be allowed only a single true sex, and the medical doctor would be the determiner or even the creator of it. Sex would now be consciously and literally constructed by the surgeon.

So we now flash forward. Since the work of John Money and his colleagues at Johns Hopkins in the 1950s, expert clinicians' understanding has been that, if children are to develop stable gender identities (and by consequence be happy and mentally healthy), they must have "correct" looking genitalia. Money's theory holds that (1) all children, intersexed and non-intersexed, are psychosexually neutral at birth, and (2) you can therefore make virtually any child either gender as long as you make the sexual anatomy reasonably believable.[9]

In one way this is the extreme opposite of the Victorian philosophy, which could be thought of as understanding sexual identity purely as a matter of "nature" (flesh and bones). Money's approach assumes nurture is the way you get to sexual identity, or what he would call gender identity. But in other ways this approach is still rather like the Victorian philosophy: it assumes doctors should be the determiners of sexual identity; it still takes the body as key; it cannot conceive of allowing a hermaphroditic identity.

Following the wide dispersal of Money's theory of gender identity development, people born intersexed are now typically subject as children to "normalizing" surgeries and hormone treatments. The general rule is this: If a child is born intersexed and has a Y chromosome, his phallus will be carefully examined. If it looks like a believable penis to the doctors, or if they think they can make it look like what they think a penis should look like, the child will be assigned the boy gender. Doctors will examine this child at regular intervals and work—using surgical and endocrinological technologies—to make him look like a "true" boy. If his phallus is less than 2.5 centimeters (1 inch) stretched at birth, however, most specialist clinicians will assign this child the girl gender, and use surgery and hormone treatments to make the patient look like what the doctors think girls should look like.

If a child is born intersexed and without a Y chromosome, doctors will assign that child the girl gender. If her clitoris is longer than 1 centimeter stretched at birth, surgeons will seek to surgically reduce it because they think it will bother the child's parents and interfere with bonding and gender identity formation. If she does not have a vagina that is, in the doctors' opinion, big enough for penetration with a penis, she will have surgery for that. Hormone treatments will eventually be used, if necessary, to get her breasts to grow, and so on.

Since the overarching rule of this system is "avoid psychological confusion about the patient's gender identity," doctors often do not tell intersexuals and their parents all that the doctors know, lest information about intersexuality confuse or complicate the family's understanding of gender. All of the professional energy is aimed at producing a physically "right" girl or boy who, presumably, the parents will then be able to raise in an unambiguous way. At the end of it all, the process is supposed to result in a well-adjusted (happy and behaviorally unambiguous) heterosexual (sleeping with people assigned the other gender) adult who complies with ongoing medical treatments (like hormone therapy), who has a fine relationship with her family, and who doesn't know she was born intersexed.

Until very recently, this practice was apparently considered—by those who knew of it—beneficent and not worth questioning. Of course, few did know of it, because intersexuality was considered rare and touchy, perhaps even taboo. Lately, however, ethicists, clinicians, and intersexuals themselves have begun to doubt the dominant clinical paradigm.

A RAPID SHIFT

Indeed, chapter 12 in this volume by Bruce Wilson and William Reiner argues that there is now taking place a paradigm shift in intersex management—from the older techno-centric treatment paradigm to a newer, ethically informed, patient-centered paradigm. Wilson and Reiner, both clinicians who work with intersexed children, argue that the older treatment model is fundamentally unsound—that it lacks empirical support and that it contradicts fundamental medical ethical principles, including "first, do no harm."

Without a doubt, the speed with which the intersex scene has been changing during this decade seems to indicate a major paradigm shift. I will add to this volume's contributors' stories my own anecdotal "postcard from the paradigm shift": A few months ago, as I was in the midst of working on this volume, I gave a talk about intersexuality at a university. My audience was diverse and included many people from outside the university system, and so I kept my presentation pretty basic. About half-way through, I showed a three-minute clip from the activist video *Hermaphrodites Speak!* [10] and contrasted this with a three-minute introductory segment from a surgery training film entitled *Surgical Reconstruction of Ambiguous Genitalia in Female Children.* [11] ("Female children" means children assigned the female gender.)

A few days after my talk, a woman in her early twenties who had been in attendance contacted me to ask me more questions about intersexuality. I'll call her Sarah. Over the course of our conversation, Sarah volunteered the information that she has a very large clitoris. She said that, though she had never been diagnosed as intersexed, she had always had a feeling that she had better hide her unusual anatomy from doctors, and had managed to do so remarkably successfully—and, after seeing the surgery video, she was glad she had. She told me she never really thought about how odd it might be that she uses her clitoris to penetrate her partner's vagina. I had mentioned in my presentation that while a large clitoris is not a medical problem—it just looks and feels different—it might indicate an underlying metabolic danger. Sarah wanted to know if she should be concerned for her health. She remembered vaguely a "hernia" operation from childhood, and now wondered if that had really been exploratory surgery to see if she had testicles.

Four years ago, in 1995, had I given this talk I would have used only pathologized images of intersexuals. No non-pathologizing images of living intersexuals (like those in this book and in *Hermaphrodites Speak!*) were available to me. As a consequence, Sarah might have been too ashamed to talk with me afterwards—indeed, I might have inadvertently made her feel positively freakish. (Heaven only knows what she or her partner would have concluded about her from my original "curiosity shop" talks on this subject.)

In 1995, had Sarah come and told me what she did, I would have actually been skeptical that she was telling me the truth. All evidence to the contrary, I still thought of intersexuality as quite rare, and frankly I had so bought into the medical textbook image of intersex that I would have had trouble believing that this articulate, three-dimensional woman could really be intersexed. (I realized recently that I had long been afraid to meet intersexuals because I figured subconsciously that when they walked up to me they would all be in black-and-white, nude, with their eyes blacked out, standing up next to a big measuring stick. What a shock it was when I realized that they look pretty much like the rest of us when you meet them at an airport, a coffee shop, or a university.)

Most significantly, in 1995 I would not have known where to refer Sarah for help. I did not know of any doctors I could trust not to cause her emotional and maybe physical pain. In spite of the fact that in 1990 Suzanne Kessler published an excellent critique of the medical management of intersex,[12] I had yet to find a physician who saw a problem with the dominant treatment system. I would have been afraid that what few support groups existed would be too nascent to really help her.

But in 1998, I could and did believe Sarah when she told me about her anatomy. Anne Fausto-Sterling has found that the frequency of intersex states is significantly higher than has generally been appreciated,[13] and I've finally come around to the data. I can now tell people with virtual certainty that we have all, in the course of our lives, met one intersexual (and probably many more). Naturally the frequency among my audiences must be even higher than the population at large; I expect to find intersexuals at about every other talk I give. Before Sarah, I had already met two other women who managed to go through life with big clitorises, so I knew that could happen. (Incidentally, all three have no interest in surgical reduction.) So I did not run away frightened from Sarah, and I did not tell her she was delusional or naive.

In 1998, I could and did refer Sarah to a select few physicians whom I could trust not to treat her with a pejorative attitude, bald voyeurism, minced words, or unwanted "corrections." I also could and did refer her to several vibrant support groups who could put her in touch with people who shared her experiences, people who could give her insight into her life history, her identity, and her future. I could send her to Suzanne

Kessler's excellent new book, *Lessons from the Intersexed.*[14] A network of helpers was in place to catch Sarah as she fell into the realization of this new identity. So, as I worked on this volume, I helped guide her through the first stages of self-discovery and realized with amazement how much the world has changed for intersexuals in just four years.[15]

PROBLEMS WITH THE DOMINANT MODEL

In conversations I have had with them, some surgeons have argued that we ought not to hastily throw out the older Age of Surgery model of intersex management for a new model. They say we first need evidence that the older model has failed and that a different model would work better. Four responses come to mind.

First, there is no real evidence that the older model works. As several of the contributors in this volume note (and as I and others have noted previously),[16] what few outcome studies there have been of intersex management have basically focused on how good the specific surgical repair turned out. In other words, we know a little about which kind of vaginoplasty results in less stenosis (scarring up), but we know almost nothing about how the women who received those vaginoplasties as girls have fared psychologically or sexually. This in spite of the fact that the older approach is premised on an understanding of intersex as a psychosocial problem. Like Wilson and Reiner, in chapter 16, Justine Marut Schober, a pediatric urological surgeon who works with intersexed children, sounds a strong note of caution and expresses concern over the long-term use of a treatment model that lacks supporting data.

In chapter 17, Kenneth Kipnis and Milton Diamond argue that this lack of follow-up studies is scandalously irresponsible; they call for cessation of unconsented surgeries until broad-based follow-up studies are done. Kipnis and Diamond also allude to evidence that the theoretical basis for the older model may well be fundamentally flawed; they cite cases and studies that suggest that children are *not* born psychosexually neutral and infinitely malleable in terms of gender formation.

Relatedly, the second response to the "keep the older model for awhile" argument is this: We do have some evidence that the older model has failed a large number of patients. Some of that is provided here, especially in parts 2 and 3. Kipnis and Diamond follow up on the famous Joan-John case. Sherri Groveman, a woman with androgen insensitivity syndrome (AIS) who leads a support group for AIS women, provides an eloquent essay explaining the dangers of doctors' withholding the whole truth from intersexed patients in chapter 2. She includes stories from AIS women to give us some sense of what it is like to have a key element of your identity shaped by medical professionals. In an essay premiering her original research, Sharon Preves, a sociologist, summarizes interviews she recently conducted with 40 adults born intersexed. She finds evidence that certain features of the older treatment paradigm—including unconsented surgeries and withholding information from patients—directly undermine the goal of producing a happy and healthy patient. Preves argues that intersex clinical treatment needs to be reworked to a point where it meets the clinicians' intentions of positive psychological outcomes.

In her chapter, Cheryl Chase quotes parents at wits' end with regard to failed "corrective" surgeries performed on their sons' penises. She questions surgeons' claims that most intersex surgeries leave patients with "normal" looking genitalia and good sexual sensation. Chase throws into doubt the efficacy and safety of current-day surgeries, and while Chase's critique is at the expert level, it doesn't take an expert to realize that most clitoral reduction surgeries will, by their very nature, reduce clitoral sensation.

Third, while it would be assuring to have long-term studies that show us that an alternative model works better than the older model, given enormous variation in nature and nurture, how could adequate controls ever be put into place for such a comparative study? As Wilson and Reiner also point out, even if we could design such a study, we would have to wait decades for the results, and in the meantime a large number of children would be subject to a medical model more and more people have concluded is unethical.

This then brings us to the fourth response to the "hold the older line for awhile" argument: Even if we had evidence that the older treatment paradigm works most of the time—which we certainly don't—we would still have to face the fact that it violates basic ethical principles now widely accepted in all realms except the treatment of children born intersexed.[17] Many of the following articles discuss this in depth, so I will just summarize the point here.

TRUTH-TELLING

The older model necessitates a basic deception. Parents are, at least in most cases, not told that the treatment model is not proven to work, is based on a peculiar theory of gender identity formation, and is increasingly widely criticized. Intersexed children, as they grow older, are kept in the dark about their conditions, even though they usually know something about them is different. (It is hard not to feel that way when doctors keep examining your genitals.) In no other realm in medicine do doctors regularly argue for active, nearly wholesale deception.

INFORMED CONSENT

The absence of full disclosure about the questionable theoretical basis of the practice and its lack of empirical support means that parents and later intersexuals themselves cannot be said to be giving informed consent. The fact that many intersexuals are not told (even when they ask) their diagnoses means they are not informed at the most basic level. Withholding of diagnoses also prevents them from researching their own condition and treatment and finding peer support.

BENEFICENCE

The older model, while designed to be beneficent, appears in many cases to actually harm intersexed children and their families by treating them as pathological and then failing to fully educate them, support them with psychological counseling by trained professionals, or refer them to peer support groups.

AUTONOMY

Intersexed people have their autonomy violated because their doctors and parents are allowed to make decisions about how their genitals should look. While intersex may signal an underlying metabolic danger, intersexed genitals are not diseased and do not have to be treated as pathological. Cosmetic surgeries are performed without the subject's consent because of adults' discomfort with intersexuality. Robert Crouch notes in his contribution that the treatment of intersex has been more about "us"—non-intersexuals—than them. These surgeries risk the subjects' sexual pleasure, health, and fertility. Several of the contributors to this volume argue that it is unethical to use such risky "cosmetic" genital surgeries on anyone who does not herself consent to them.

TOWARD THE AGE OF CONSENT

In his classic study of paradigm shifts, Thomas Kuhn showed that major theoretical shifts tend to occur not because the evidence for a newer theory outweighs the evidence for an older one, but rather because core beliefs change.[18] The shift in intersex management now taking place follows this model. Clinicians are beginning to abandon the older model of intersex management not because we have vast quantities of data to show that a newer model works better, but because medicine as a whole has moved toward patient-centered, ethically principled care. The fact that intersex management has taken so long to catch up can only be due to the fact that we treat "abnormality"—especially the sexual sort—as a special case.

While the following articles differ in some fine points, this general new model for intersex management arises from them:

PROVIDE PSYCHOLOGICAL SUPPORT TO PARENTS

When a child is born intersexed (or diagnosed as intersexed prenatally), parents should immediately be offered psychological support. We know in part from Joan Ablon's research on families dealing with achondroplasia that parents of children born with unusual anatomies typically undergo a grieving process in which they grieve the loss of the anticipated "normal" child.[19] Parents of intersexuals therefore need to be referred to professional counselors who understand grief, parenting, and the complexities of gender. They also need to be referred to peer support groups so that they receive assurance from other parents that their feelings and concerns are normal and manageable.[20] From my conversations with intersexuals and their parents, it is clear that the role of counselor should not be left to an endocrinologist, urologist, geneticist, or surgeon.

ASSIGN A GENDER

All children—no matter how intersexed—can and should be assigned a male or female gender. This consists of physicians helping parents understand which gender assignment makes the most sense (that is, which is likely to be the one the child will ultimately identify with). Will some intersexed children assigned, say, the boy gender decide later they are girls? Yes. And so will some non-intersexed boys. Hard as it is to accept, we have to recognize that *every* gender assignment is preliminary, whether the child being assigned a gender is intersexed or non-intersexed.

PROVIDE NON-PATHOLOGIZED IMAGES

Intersexuals, their parents, medical students, residents, genetic counselors, and so on need to be provided with non-pathologized images of intersexuals, or they will inevitably see intersexuality as deeply pathological. These images should be of all types—textual, visual, face-to-face, and so on. This book provides a place to start. Support groups are the best sources for more of these resources.[21]

DELAY COSMETIC SURGERIES AND HORMONE TREATMENTS

Medical problems of intersex children should obviously be addressed. Some of those problems will require surgery, for example when a child is born with a urinary tract that drains in such a way as to lead to repeated infections. But surgeries and hormone treatments designed simply to change the look of genitalia should not be done unless explicitly requested by the patient him/herself. At that time, the patient should be informed of the risks of the treatment options, and should be provided with long-term results of the options. How old should a child have to be before she or he can be said to be capable of informed consent? This is obviously a difficult and persistent question in medical ethics, but the fact that it is a difficult question does not mean that the question should be subverted by allowing risky and unnecessary surgeries on children before they can consent.

LIMIT STRESSFUL CLINICAL DISPLAYS

Virtually all the of intersexed people who write in this volume stress the trauma caused by being repeatedly "put on display" for medical students, residents, and attending physicians. While medical professionals need to be educated about intersex by seeing real cases, they must also recognize the psychological harm done to intersexed patients—especially children—when they are repeatedly obligated to make their genitalia available for visual and physical examination by students and physicians. Clinicians will need to develop ways to educate without making intersexed patients feel freakish and violated.

PROVIDE PSYCHOLOGICAL SUPPORT TO THE CHILD

Intersexed children face special psychosocial problems. Everyone agrees on this. Therefore intersexed children should be provided with pediatric counselors and peer support groups. Their concerns, fears, and questions should be answered honestly.

RECOGNIZE INTERSEXUALS AS EXPERTS

A major failure of the older model has arisen from the failure to recognize intersexed people as experts of their own experiences. A patient-centered model of intersex would take seriously intersexuals' opinions and critiques of various treatments. This would include long-term studies with all intersexed patients to determine which kinds of treatments helped or hurt them.

The reader will see that the following articles mostly agree on this overall strategy. I would like to note that I worked to find an author who would defend the older treatment model of intersex. My requests for contributions from proponents of the older model were met with silence or the apology that potential contributors lacked the time to write for this volume.

BEYOND THE FIVE SEXES

When I speak about intersexuality, people often express to me the suspicion that science will eventually sort out this whole sex thing, and then we'll be able to say for sure what makes a male, what a female, and what a hermaphrodite. But such a hope is chasing after ghosts. In a groundbreaking article in 1993, Anne Fausto-Sterling argued that we need to recognize that there are five sexes in the human population: females, males, female pseudo-hermaphrodites, male pseudo-hermaphrodites, and true hermaphrodites.[22] But we know now that this very division into "five sexes" developed in 1896 as just one more cultural attempt to keep the threat of the hermaphrodite at bay. The fact that the term "true hermaphrodite" is still reserved for people born with both ovarian and testicular tissue is just a Victorian hangover.

So what is a true hermaphrodite? We can't really say. Anatomy is never going to tell us for sure what sex is all about or who is really an intersexual. As humans we decide that. We decide who gets to count as a male, what you have to have or do to count as a female, and what happens to you if you get labeled intersexed. Indeed, sociological and anthropological research indicates that we don't all even think of "man" and "woman" the same, no less intersex. In other times and other places, some people have even held up the hermaphrodite as an ideal, or as a sacred identity. (Robert Crouch discusses some of these alternative visions in his chapter.)

All theory aside, in real life sexual variation blends imperceptibly one kind into the next. The treatment of people born with notably unusual anatomies isn't going to be resolved by the discovery of some gene that reveals the ultimate nature of sexual identity. John Money was right in at least one way—we make it up as we go along, and yes, the body does matter—but in ways that continue to surprise and vary from person to person. In the end, all intersexuals are now asking is to be treated according to the same ethical principles as everybody else. This volume seeks to explore what that would mean.

ACKNOWLEDGMENT

This chapter first appeared in *The Journal of Clinical Ethics* 9, no. 4 (Winter 1998); © 1998 by *The Journal of Clinical Ethics*; used with permission. Photo used with the permission of Aron Sousa.

NOTES

1. A.D. Dreger, *Hermaphrodites and the Medical Invention of Sex* (Cambridge, Mass.: Harvard University Press, 1998), 25-26.

2. For an elaboration of this history, see ibid., chapter 5.

3. Ibid., 119-26.

4. T. Tuffier and A. Lapointe, "L'Hermaphrodisme: Ses variétés et ses conséquences pour la pratique médicale (d'après un cas personnel)," *Revue de gynécologie et de chirurgie abdominale* 17 (1911): 209-68, at 256.

5. For more on the motivations for the Gonadal Definition, see Dreger, *Hermaphrodites and the Medical Invention of Sex*, note 1 above, pp. 150-54.

6. W.B. Bell, "Hermaphroditism," *Liverpool Medico-Chirurgical Journal* 35 (1915): 272-92, at 291.

7. Ibid., 277.

8. Ibid., 292. Incidentally, this is the first use I can find of the word "gender" in medical literature on hermaphroditism.

9. For a review and critique of Money's work, see C. Chase, "Hermaphrodites with Attitude: Mapping the Emergence of Intersex Political Activism," *GLQ: A Journal of Gay and Lesbian Studies* 4, no. 2 (1998): 189-211. Also see A. Fausto-Sterling, "How to Build a Man," in *Science and Homosexualities*, ed. V.A. Rosario (New York: Routledge, 1997), 219-25.

10. *Hermaphrodites Speak!* Intersex Society of North America (ISNA), 26 minutes, 1997, videocassette. Copies may be obtained from ISNA, P.O. Box 31791, San Francisco, Calif. 94131; website < www.isna.org >.

11. R.S. Hurwitz, H. Applebaum, and S. Muenchow, *Surgical Reconstruction of Ambiguous Genitalia in Female Children*, ACS/USSC Educational Library, no. ACS-1613, 21 minutes, 1990, videocassette. Copies may be obtained from Cine-Med, 127 Main St. North, P.O. Box 745, Woodbury, Conn. 06798; telephone (800) 633-0004.

12. S.J. Kessler, "The Medical Construction of Gender: Case Management of Intersexed Infants," *Signs* 16 (1990): 3-26.

13. M. Blackless et al., "How Sexually Dimorphic Are We?" *American Journal of Human Biology* (forthcoming). On the difficulty of calculating the frequency of intersexuality, see Dreger, *Hermaphrodites and the Medical Invention of Sex,* see note 1 above, pp. 40-43.

14. S.J. Kessler, *Lessons from the Intersexed* (Piscataway, N.J.: Rutgers University Press, 1998).

15. For a summary of this recent history, see Chase, "Hermaphrodites with Attitude," see note 9 above.

16. See A.D. Dreger, "'Ambiguous Sex'—or Ambivalent Medicine? Ethical Issues in the Treatment of Intersexuality," *Hastings Center Report* 28, no. 3 (May-June 1998): 24-35; see also J.M. Schober, "Feminizing Genitoplasty for Intersex," in *Pediatric Surgery and Urology: Long Term Outcomes,* ed. M.D. Stringer et al. (London: W.B. Saunders, 1998), 549-58.

17. For more on this argument, see Dreger, "'Ambiguous Sex'—or Ambivalent Medicine?" see note 16 above.

18. S. Kuhn, *The Structure of Scientific Revolutions* (Chicago: University of Chicago Press, 1996, 1962).

19. J. Ablon, "Ambiguity and Difference: Families with Dwarf Children," *Social Science and Medicine* 30, no. 8 (1990): 879-87.

20. The easiest way to locate intersex support groups is through the home page of the Intersex Society of North America, see note 10 above.

21. Ibid.

22. A. Fausto-Sterling, "The Five Sexes," *The Sciences* 33 (1993): 20-25.

2

The Hanukkah Bush:
Ethical Implications in the Clinical
Management of Intersex

Sherri A. Groveman

As a young child of a conservative, but unobservant, Jewish house-hold, I viewed Christmas as being about the large, aromatic firs and spruces adorning my friends' apartments, decorated with dazzling ornaments and surrounded by a profusion of foil-wrapped packages. Hanukkah, by contrast, was embodied in our home by only a small menorah on our window sill. Is it any wonder that I begged, pleaded, and cajoled my parents for a Christmas tree? Wisely, they would not relent.

Soon I discovered that the parents of some Jewish friends had insti-tuted a custom of "Hanukkah bushes," which, to any honest observer, were clearly Christmas trees in drag. Seeing one for the first time it felt fake, hollow, half of something but all of nothing. My friends' parents, uncomfortable about their minority status, had been co-opted by the overwhelming pressure to make life "easier" for their children by dilut-ing their heritage while assimilating to the dominant culture.

With the benefit of hindsight, I am glad my parents did not yield to such pressure even as I regret they did not do more to educate me about my roots. Having now learned the history of my religion, I have discov-ered all that is rich and precious about Hanukkah, dissipating any desire for a Christmas tree. My "Hanukkah bush" friends, by contrast, derive no such meaning from the Festival of Lights, but at the same time feel like frauds if they lay claim to actual Christmas trees. Did their parents' response to societal pressure, though well-intentioned to help these chil-dren "fit in," simply leave my friends incapable of functioning comfortably in either world? Can the same be said of doctors who importune parents to manage their intersex children with surgery and secrets?

I might mention, as a footnote to this parable, that the population of Jews in the world is no larger than the population of intersex persons. Thus, I suppose it is fortunate that pediatric endocrinologists are not the stewards of the world's religions, because with the same rationale they use to support surgery and secrecy in managing intersex—that is, that it is unfair to leave children's ambiguous genitals in their natural state, or even openly acknowledge to them that they are intersexed, because this will render them outcasts to the majority of society—these doctors might argue that it is unfair to obligate children to live with a religion shared by only a tiny fraction of the world's population. As a practical matter, of course, religious tolerance is an accepted norm in our society, whereas doctors perceive something inherently intolerable about intersex.

Intersex is a subject near and dear to my heart (and other parts of my anatomy). But it is also my personal history inflected by the burden of having lived almost all of my 40 years with the shame, secrecy, and isolation that are an inevitable by-product of how my case was managed by the medical profession.

I have complete androgen insensitivity syndrome (AIS), which is characterized by XY chromosomes and testes, but a complete inability, due to an androgen receptor defect, of the body to respond to the testosterone produced by the testes. Unable to virilize, my body, by preordination, simply developed along a female path. In my case, this was discovered 10 days after my birth, when my pediatrician noticed a swelling in my groin, suggesting a hernia. Exploratory surgery performed at two weeks revealed the presence of what seemed to be a testis. When the lab report confirmed this, my parents were told that it was medically necessary for them to consent to immediate gonadectomy. Lacking any better insight, they of course gave their consent.

In fact, there was no urgent medical necessity; my testes could have remained safely intact until puberty, at which time they should have been removed to prevent any risk of cancer. But I strongly suspect that there were pressing "psychological" necessities for their removal in infancy: (1) my doctors' desire to rid me of any vestige of a male anatomy and render my body "congruent"; (2) the equal desire to avoid the need at puberty to explain the nature of the surgery that would have to be performed, raising questions the doctors did not want to have to answer; and (3) shards of a superstitious fear that, despite what medicine knew in 1958 about "testicular feminization" (as it was then called), I might somehow virilize if my troublesome gonads were left intact.

Unlike Hanukkah, where my parents were sufficiently inculcated with the traditions of their religion to inoculate them against the pressure to conform to the dominant messages surrounding them, my parents are not, alas, intersexed, and so to learn the "culture" of what this meant to their child they had to rely on doctors to translate the language and meaning of words such as "chromosomes" and "gonads" and "pseudohermaphrodite." Unfortunately, like most doctors even today, my doctors were steeped in a tradition that viewed intersexuality as a tragedy—a mistake of nature to be corrected, to the maximum extent possible, by medicine. This culture had been handed down to them without any concern for the long-term outcome of the recipients of such treatment protocols. Thus, they became self-appointed tour guides to a foreign country when they themselves had not bothered to ever communicate with the natives.

My experience over the past three years assisting families affected by AIS informs me that the most critical variable to achieving a better outcome for intersex patients is not surgical management followed up with platitudes and half-truths, but instead is the provision of resources for parents to be thoroughly educated about what intersex is, and to work through any anxiety or guilt they feel about having an intersex child. When parents are able to communicate their comfort and acceptance, the child's self-esteem can develop from a solid foundation. When parents are, by contrast, apprehensive, fearful, or ignorant about intersex, their child is left to flounder in a sea of confusion without support. Regrettably medicine has seen fit to "correct" what is between the child's legs while offering limited educational assistance and psychological support to either the child or her/his family.

Indeed, the sole instruction my parents received from my endocrinologists was one of "damage control," calculated to confirm a solid image that I was their daughter in the same breath that doctors enjoined them that they should not disclose my true diagnosis to anyone, least of all me. While informing my parents that I was "just like a normal female," my doctors offered no suggestions other than fabrication about how they should help me cope with the reality of having XY chromosomes and testes while lacking ovaries, a uterus, fallopian tubes, or fertility.

Fortuitously, my surgeon failed to diagnose that I have a vagina incapable of intromission; had he done so he likely would have suggested vaginoplasty, a procedure that continues to be recommended in childhood to this day, despite its nearly 80 percent failure rate when performed prior to adolescence. Had I had been born with more ambiguous looking genitals, the solution offered would have been more surgery, most likely to make my genitals appear "female," even at the expense of diminishing sexual sensation. Cultural imperative, masquerading as medical necessity, would have made such additional surgeries inevitable.

I spent my adolescence filled with shame, though I was never told the true details of my diagnosis. My trauma was needlessly compounded by my doctor's stony silence while examining me, and his asking me to lie naked on an examining table so that teams of interns and residents could inspect my genitals. Such experiences themselves, far more than the true facts I later learned about the nature of AIS, instilled a sense of freakishness that I have only recently shaken. It is, however, disheartening to hear that similar treatment of intersex adolescents continues to this day.

Ultimately, I unearthed the truth about having AIS in a medical school library when I was 20 by researching the possible causes for my primary amenorrhea and lack of pubic hair. It is disorienting when you have always considered yourself female to learn that you have XY chromosomes and once had testes. It is equally disorienting when you have always considered yourself loved and cared for to discover that your parents and doctors have lied and left you to your own devices to discover this truth.

I appreciate that because I am 40 years old my treatment protocol was a product of 1960s thinking. I am frightened, however, that as we approach the turn of the millennium conventional medical treatment continues to endorse a nearly identical protocol. Doctors continue to debate the patient's right to know the truth, seemingly oblivious to the idea that they do not "own" the patient's medical information. This conspiracy of silence stems from the same root as the continuing protocol to surgically alter intersex infants' anatomies—an inability to see intersex as anything other than shameful and pathologic. This, in turn, is communicated to the parents, whom I believe would be far less traumatized by the reality of intersex if they weren't receiving such negative cues from doctors.

Regrettably, doctors fail to offer appropriate psychological support to parents or even communicate that the capacity to give and receive love is a function of the size of one's heart, not the size or appearance of one's genitals. Yet this capacity for healthy relationships is threatened at best, and more typically destroyed altogether, through the toxic mixture of silence and surgery that is offered up as the only "solution" to the child's intersex "problem."

In the aftermath of such surgery, doctors behave as though the "problem" has been cured ("you used to be intersexed but we fixed it")—as though being intersexed were a historic detail of the patient's life. Unfortunately, this too is communicated to the parents, who, in turn, assume that there is no need to offer their child a safe place to mourn and grieve what has occurred, or to help their child ascribe meaning to being intersexed. Often the parents are sufficiently uncomfortable and guilt-ridden about the whole affair that they are highly motivated to accept the doctor's revisionist history of the child's intersex state. Thus, the child has endured a personal holocaust while having to remain mute.

I believe, based upon my experiences overseeing the U.S. branch of the AIS Support Group, attending 10 AIS Support Group meetings in the U.S. and the U.K., and getting to know more than 100 intersex people, ranging in age from two months to 73 years, that under the best of circumstances learning the truth about being intersexed can be temporarily traumatic. But not knowing the truth culminates in experiences that are almost universally tragic. With limited, inaccurate information, and in the face of an overarching sense of shame, the mind conjures a parade of horribles far worse than any truth. Indeed, of the more than 60 women with AIS whom I personally know, I have not heard of a single instance where someone has reported that it was worse to know the truth than to live with lies.

Fortunately, many pediatric endocrinologists are endorsing the approach of truthful disclosure at the same time that they are revisiting the wisdom of surgical management of intersex. Apart from the ethical implications of a protocol rooted in dissimulation, the paradigm of deceit is, quite simply, shortsighted. The reports of women affiliated with the AIS Support Group reveal that patients are driven to learn what it is about themselves that seems to cause a palpable silence whenever they are examined by doctors or broach the subject of their childhood/adolescent gonadectomies. To that end, some members of our support group became expert in reading their medical charts upside down, while others inspected their files when their doctors momentarily left the examining room.

But there are even more unusual, and often painful, ways this information is obtained. Some members report the "dreaded" information spilling out in the heat of arguments with stepparents or siblings. One woman in our U.K. group literally discovered she had AIS by buying a house. She applied for a mortgage which required that she provide proof of good health. To do so she had to sign a medical release. She had never been told she had AIS—just that she had an "ovarian" problem and couldn't have children, but that this had no bearing on her health. She innocently signed the release. A few weeks later her mortgage company called her and said, "Everything is fine but we need to know what this 'androgen insensitivity' thing is all about."

It is important to note that the significance of truth-telling has increased with the advent of intersex support groups, such as the AIS Support Group, the Intersex Society of North America, and the Coalition for Intersex Support Advocacy and Education. These support groups provide a culture for intersexuals as well as validation of feelings; they offer enormous psychological relief for parents of intersex children, as well as intersex adolescents and adults.

To illustrate, in the case of AIS, many parents are understandably concerned about how they will communicate to their daughters that they have XY chromosomes; these parents are typically uncomfortable about this fact themselves. However, at a recent meeting of the AIS Support Group our members decided to take a photograph with the adult women with AIS, and the fathers of children with AIS, forming "Y's" with their arms while the mothers of such children crossed their arms to form "X's." The ability to defuse tension about "the chromosome thing" quite visibly allowed these parents to feel more comfortable and accepting of the entire issue.

Perhaps it is fitting that I have used a holiday theme in this article. For it was the day after Christmas in 1994 when I first discovered, while researching in a medical school library, that an AIS Support Group had recently been founded in the U.K. No gift I will receive in this lifetime will ever be as precious to me as discovering that information. My subsequent involvement with the support group has, remarkably, allowed me to view having AIS as a blessing—after all, if I didn't have AIS I would not have developed into the woman I believe God and nature intended me to be. This was certainly not the outcome my doctors would have predicted on a chilly September day when they removed my gonads and implored my parents never to tell me the truth. The miracle of life, however, is that we can evolve; I hope that this same miracle can touch those who will be privileged to care for the intersex children born while this article was being read.

ACKNOWLEDGMENT

This chapter first appeared in *The Journal of Clinical Ethics* 9, no. 4 (Winter 1998); © 1998 by *The Journal of Clinical Ethics*; used with permission.

3

Betwixt and Between:
The Past and Future of Intersexuality

Robert A. Crouch

INTRODUCTION

Though gender pervades our daily lives—used, as it is, to designate both ourselves and others as man or woman, boy or girl—it does so in a curiously tacit manner. As Judith Lorber notes, talking about gender is much like "a fish talking about water."[1] Like water to the fish, gender (like sex) is at once the medium within which we live our lives and at the same time part of the taken-for-granted, background assumptions that are rarely questioned. Both sex and gender seem simply to be *there*— natural, immutable, dual, and tightly coupled.

Yet the certainty with which one can claim that there are only two sexes and only two *corresponding* genders is often unclear. Simply put, "sex is a shaky foundation,"[2] and with instabilities in sex can often come instabilities in gender—though, as the case of transvestitism convincingly demonstrates, the tight correspondence between sex and gender can easily be upset even when sex is stable. The uncertainty regarding the tight correspondence between sex and gender is perhaps best illustrated when a child is born with an intersexed condition; that is, with external genitalia that are "ambiguous" and neither clearly female nor male. It is precisely such a moment, when an intersexed child is born and the medical team and family cannot name it as male or female, that our system of sex categorization is called into question[3] and we are forced to re-examine many of our previously certain, though taken-for-granted, background beliefs.

The recognition that one's background cultural beliefs might not be immutable can cause anxiety. Jared Diamond writes that confrontations with gender ambiguity provoke "nervous squirming in almost all of us"[4] and the same can be said of sexual ambiguity. This is so, as Lorber writes, because "Gender signs and signals are so ubiquitous that we usually fail to note them—unless they are missing or ambiguous. Then we are uncomfortable until we have successfully placed the other person in a gender status; otherwise, *we* feel socially dislocated."[5] But this is precisely what disconcerts: the "problem" with ambiguous sex and gender, and by implication with intersexed persons, seems to be a problem with the *rest of us*.

STANDARD OF CARE: DISCOVERY TO CREATION

An examination of the recent medical literature reveals a similar social discomfort with intersexuality among modern medical practitioners, one perhaps not unfairly described as often bordering on alarm. Healthcare professionals who write about intersexuality and its treatment do so as if following the same script: "The birth of an infant with ambiguous genitalia is a medical and psychosocial emergency . . . ";[6] "Gender assignment . . . must be considered a psychosocial emergency . . . carried out against time in terms of days, even hours";[7] "Ambiguous external genitalia of the neonate is generally considered a medical and social emergency . . . ";[8] "The birth of an infant with ambiguous genitalia is a social and potentially medical emergency";[9] and so on.[10] What is striking about these excerpts is their description of the birth of an intersex child as being a *psychosocial* or *social* emergency. While intersexuality *might* be a sign of a serious underlying medical condition, which physicians should always treat when medically necessary,[11] such medical emergencies are distinct from the social emergencies being referred to in these passages. Why, then, the social emergency?

When an intersexed child is born, the parents and the medical team are faced with a question: Is this a boy or a girl? The gender is unclear because the child's sex is thought to be unclear. The child who cannot be placed by physicians into one of two available sex categories is thus deemed to be in urgent need of medical attention, and is to that extent pathologized. Such pathologizing of intersexed children is facilitated by current medical thinking on the matter. Unlike the previous century's preoccupation with the gonads and with the *discovery* of a person's "true sex,"[12] the view that dominates medical practice today is one that moves away from the old model in two ways: first, there is a clear emphasis placed upon the future *gender* rather than the sex of the child; and, second, there is a more explicit awareness that the medical intervention sets out not to discover, but to *create* a child of a certain gender. This aspect of gender creation is nicely captured in the title of a recent paper by Anne Fausto-Sterling: "How to Build a Man."[13]

As Wilson and Reiner note in this volume, the current management philosophy is premised on two largely unexamined, but deeply held principles that have retained their clinical centrality since first promulgated by John Money and his colleagues in the 1950s.[14] First, individuals are hypothesized to be psychosexually neutral at birth and thought to remain so for about two years; and, second, one's healthy psychosexual development is presumed to depend on the "normal" appearance of one's genitals. This second principle, implicitly tying genital appearance to gender role and identity, encompasses both how the person perceives his or her own sex and gender, and how he or she is perceived by others, as man or woman, boy or girl. Physicians, therefore, have proceeded as if the sex (hence, future gender) of the intersexed child can be selected, regardless of the child's genetic complement, and have based this sex and gender selection upon the possible future appearance of the child's genitalia. In other words, sex and gender assignment depends on what surgeons believe they can *make of* the genitals they have to *work with*. Once sex is selected for the child, it is recommended that no doubt should be expressed by the parents, or others around the child, as to the child's sex of assignment. And, to complete the script, it is advised that the sex should not be changed after two years of age.[15]

In practice, this means that in the case of the male pseudohermaphrodite, if physicians judge that they can make the phallus large enough through androgen therapy and surgery to be an "adequate" and "functional" penis, then they decide that the child is male; if they judge otherwise, then the phallus is reduced in size to become a "clitoris."[16] They also typically recommend, in the latter case, surgical construction of a "vagina" and hormonal therapy.[17] In the case of the female pseudohermaphrodite, if they judge it to be necessary, physicians reduce the clitoris in size and construct a "vagina" and "labia" to make the child appear more clearly female. Baldly stated, the medical team selects a gender for the child and, in so doing, explicitly endorses the view that the perception of the child's genitals is more influential than anything else in terms of gender identity formation. Given the assumed importance of the perception of the child's genitals, physicians bring the child's appearance in line with the assigned sex and thus "force" the child into one of two available sex or gender categories via surgery and hormone therapy.

The persistence of such practices would suggest an evolving body of empirical literature that, presumably, confirms Money's original hypothesis. As others in this volume have demonstrated, such a body of confirmatory (or, non-falsificatory) evidence, however, has not been forthcoming, and Money's hypothesis remains a mere hypothesis to this day. Though some practitioners simply proclaim that excellent long-term outcomes can be expected[18] and others claim, contrary to fact, that there exists a large body of evidence that confirms that sex of rearing is overriding in gender identity formation,[19] most are honest that no such follow-up data exists and that treatment decisions are highly speculative.[20] Indeed, as one medical team put it in an unintentionally revealing passage, "The decision for a sex change [that is, sex assignment] must not be made by one person; rather, a team of experts should be responsible, because the decision cannot be made on a firm scientific basis."[21] Treatment decisions for intersexed children have not been made on a "firm scientific basis," yet they have been made nonetheless.

CRITIQUE, NORM, UTOPIA?

What emerges from a reading of the literature surrounding the medical treatment of intersexed persons is that dubious criteria, and correspondingly questionable outcome measures, are invoked when deciding upon the child's sex assignment and when determining whether a sex assignment intervention counts as a success. Moreover, the sex assignment criteria, though explicitly having to do with the appearance of the genitals, are clearly linked to socio-cultural gender norms. With treatment choices made, as we shall see, for the most part on non-medical grounds, and given the level of emergency with which the birth of an intersexed child is met in the clinic, one cannot help but conclude that intersexed children are being pathologized by the medical professions; in other words, the variant genitals of intersexed children are invested with negative meaning by physicians with the "power to name."[22]

And name they do. A larger than typical clitoris has been variously described as "a disfiguring and embarrassing phallic structure," an "ungainly masculine enlargement," a "button of unsightly tissue," an "anatomical derangement," and an "embarrassing or offensive" phallic enlargement.[23] These descriptions reveal not strictly medical concerns but, rather, social and aesthetic ones; yet the intersexed are surgically treated with an urgency that bespeaks an underlying *medical* pathology toward which the surgery is directed *as* treatment. These aesthetic pathologies lead surgeons to perform clitoral reduction operations that sometimes fail to preserve sexual sensation and can leave such women without the ability to achieve orgasm.[24]

Similar social and aesthetic considerations are operative regarding the surgical construction of a "vagina." Since the vagina is widely regarded as merely a "passive organ,"[25] the real concern is to make sure that the vaginal opening (introitus) looks good and that it and the constructed "vagina" are of sufficient dimension to receive a penis, regardless of whether the "vagina" can be sexually responsive for the woman. Cheryl Chase, an intersexed woman whom surgeons subjected to childhood genital surgeries (including clitorectomy), reports that after her physician examined her and noted that the area where her clitoris had been was sexually unfeeling, the physician comforted her by saying, "You'll get someone to hold you nice and you'll be ok."[26] Looming in the background of all of this is a moralistic and gendered cultural script that views women as passive recipients during sex, simply there to please their sexual partners, and not themselves agents of sexual desire and feeling.

A similar cultural impetus drives the treatment of "male" intersexed children. For with these intersexed individuals, it is the size of the phallus—acting as a spatio-temporal proxy for future gender identity—that determines the sex of assignment. So powerful is the logic at work here that, should the newborn's phallus fall under a length required by the pediatric urologist, the medical team will assign that child to the female sex and surgically and hormonally erase any physical traces of maleness.[27] Indeed, one group treats the child with a micropenis as if he had no penis at all: "They must be raised as females. . . . They are doomed to life as a male without a penis,"[28] though evidence exists to the contrary.[29] Moreover, should the child have a hypospadic penis (a common condition where the urethral opening is not located at the tip of the penis),[30] surgeons will perform painful genital surgery on the child so that he may be able to urinate with a steady stream while standing up and, as one group put it, be able to show his "prowess at urinating at certain distances in competition with other boys."[31] The implicit message here is that to have a stable male sex and masculine gender identity one must first have a sufficiently large penis so that one can look like and "perform" as a male in childhood, and so that one can satisfy one's sexual partner later on, even if that means having a scarred and desensitized penis.[32] The clinical consensus on this seems to be: "Penetration in the absence of pleasure takes precedence over pleasure in the absence of penetration."[33]

Among clinicians who work with intersexed individuals, then, the motivation for treatment seems to be socio-cultural rather than medical.[34] Sex assignment decisions are based upon the appearance of the genitals and the prospects for achieving the gender role deemed "appropriate" to the newly crafted genitals. The gender of the intersexed person, as indeed with all persons, is thus both ascribed and achieved.[35] Gender is ascribed explicitly by the family and by others insofar as the child is directed into "gender-appropriate" activities (playing with dolls versus playing with tools), behaviors (attentive listener versus aggressive debater) and roles (homemaker versus professional), and is ascribed implicitly, when the child is sanctioned for "gender-inappropriate" deviations or praised for "gender-appropriate" behavior.[36] But gender is also achieved insofar as the child eventually adopts the socially available gender norms and expresses those appropriately in social space.[37] Unlike most other persons, however, intersexed children have their gender inscribed by physicians directly on the body—as Kiira Triea revealingly puts it, highlighting at the same time the way that dominant treatment regimes are much like articles of faith, "They tried to write their Gospel / on my body."[38] Via sex-making surgeries, the aim of the male or female sex inscription is to fashion genitalia of "acceptable" appearance and to ensure proper gender identity and performance.[39]

But acceptable to whom? One of the claims that I have made is that the reaction to the intersexed child reveals less about *intersexuality* than it does about a social and medical *discomfort with intersexuality*. Physicians and family members, to be sure, are not immune from the influence of prevalent socio-cultural norms and, thus, one should take care, as Carl Elliott writes, not to misleadingly ascribe to them "a conscious effort to fend off threats to a cultural order."[40] Indeed, as Kessler notes, the motive force behind the current treatment philosophy should perhaps be located in the agency of culture: "if culture demands gender, physicians will produce it, and of course, when physicians produce it, the fact that gender is 'demanded' will be hidden from everyone."[41]

Nonetheless, while healthcare workers and especially parents evince legitimate and undoubtedly justifiable concern for the intersexed child, the worry I have occurs when such solicitude crosses over into a pity for those who are considered deviant and dysfunctional. It is when intersexed persons are subject to multiple surgeries, thought of by most intersexed persons as mutilating, and when they are referred to as "unfortunate individuals"[42] who one day, it is hoped, "will meet with the sympathy they deserve,"[43] that one can see that the medical pathologizing of intersexuality must be resisted if intersexed persons are to be accorded the respect they are due. The variant genitals of intersexed children are invested with negative meaning that usually leads to a surgical intervention and an often poor outcome for the child. But it is this first step, the naming of the genitals as either "pathological," "ambiguous," on the one hand, or as "variant," on the other, that is crucial; for, while it is understandable that "something needs to be done about 'ambiguity,' . . . it is less obvious what (if anything) needs to be done about 'variability'."[44] Indeed, as Kessler remarks about the treatment of intersexuals, "Institutionalized mutilations occur because the genitals are taken too seriously. It is not that the *material* genitals are respected but that the *idea* of genitals is . . . . If we want people to respect *particular* bodies, they need to be taught to lose respect for *ideal* ones."[45] Held captive by an image of the "normal" child, surgeons sculpt the intersexed newborn's material form in pursuit of the elusive ideal.

LIMINALITY AND SOCIAL STATUS

I have maintained that the medical community regards the intersexed child as being somehow deviant and in need of medical attention and, in doing so, mirrors broader cultural norms regarding acceptable sex and gender. In this regard, the motivating reasons for the medical management of intersexed children are aesthetic and cultural, rather than medical and, I have suggested, defeasible. I would like now to look at this issue within a somewhat different framework, but in the service of the very same point, namely, that cultural reasons ground the medical management of intersexed children. This, I hope, will provide further reason to reject the present intersex management philosophy and to think about intersexuality anew.

Gender as a social category is of central importance within society; indeed, in the West, if one is neither man nor woman, then one has no social place or state to occupy. In their treatment of intersexed children, physicians concern themselves with securing a social state—a future gender role—for the child. They ask in part: given the genital appearances that can be achieved with surgery and hormone therapy, what gender role could this child most successfully occupy? Though it is the child's "ambiguous" sex that initially prompts concern, the child's future gender state drives treatment choice. Implicit in this clinical logic is the belief that the intersexed child's future social status is in jeopardy if no medical intervention is undertaken; put differently, the intersexed child will be unable to achieve a gender unless a male or female sex is ascribed and surgically inscribed on the body. To be gendered, one must first be sexed, not intersexed.

Like social class or age in certain societies at certain times, gender too structures social relations and thus counts among the statuses through which individuals are "seen" socially. In the West, gender both stratifies and structures society.[46] Though differences are arguably becoming smaller, men and women are socially and legally far from being treated equally.[47] Similarly, gender has built into it certain social possibilities (though again these are in flux); in other words, with one's gender come certain social roles that are more easily (that is, acceptably) occupied than others—for example, though it is the case empirically, it need not be true that women, far more often than men, forego paid employment to raise children full-time. The structuring function of gender is certainly more perspicuous in some societies than in others—compare certain Western societies to certain Muslim societies—but what is meant by "structure" is often the same.[48] Following anthropologist Victor Turner's account, social structure is the " 'patterned arrangements of role-sets, status-sets, and status-sequences' *consciously* recognized and regularly operative in a given society."[49] Tightly bound up with political and legal categories, social structure has a certain "cognitive quality" and is "essentially a set of classifications, a model for thinking about culture and nature and ordering one's public life."[50] It is through structure (including, but by no means limited to, gender), therefore, that we conceptualize the world.

This view of society as a "differentiated, segmented system of structural positions"[51] creates the possibility that there will be some who cannot be placed in a structural position and who thus find themselves "in the interstices of social structures."[52] This inter-structural phase, as Turner refers to it, is characterized by the *liminality* of the social actors; that is, by their ambiguity and lack of social definition.[53] Having slipped through the "network of classifications that normally locate states and positions in cultural space," liminal persons are "neither here nor there; they are betwixt and between the positions assigned and arrayed by law, custom, convention, and ceremonial."[54] Such persons are, therefore, "structurally 'dead' "[55] and, to this extent, socially problematic. For in their ambiguous state, the liminal person is made to be "an exile or a stranger, someone who, by his very existence, calls into question the whole normative order."[56]

And so it is with the intersexed child, the child who appears neither clearly male nor clearly female and is therefore at risk of becoming neither man nor woman, or so the behavior of physicians seems clearly to imply. The structural elements that are important in the case of the intersexed child are sex and gender, where these clearly structure our own society via accompanying and often defining roles and statuses. The liminal character of intersexed children is made manifest by the "social emergency" declared by physicians after their birth. This reaction of emergency occurs precisely because we lack the socio-cultural categories that enable us to so effectively conceptualize the other humans with whom we interact on a daily basis. As Turner notes, "most of us see only what we expect to see, and what we expect to see is what we are conditioned to see when we have learned the definitions and classifications of our culture. A society's secular definitions do not allow for the existence of a not-boy-not-man,"[57] as in initiation rites, nor, as Turner would probably agree, a not-boy-not-girl.

It is therefore no wonder that physicians write of intersexual social emergencies. The way that physicians deal with intersexed children suggests that such children are thought of as being inherently in a transitional state; for the non-treatment of intersexed children clearly has not been a real option. The medical management philosophy can therefore not unreasonably be seen as an attempt by physicians to transfer the intersexed child from a liminal, ambiguous state into a structured—male- or female-sexed, masculine- or feminine-gendered—state, thereby reproducing cultural norms on the body of the intersexed child. As Kessler writes, the "genital ambiguity is remedied to conform to a 'natural,' that is, culturally indisputable gender dichotomy"[58] and, to that extent I would claim, so too is the child's ambiguous social identity—his or her liminality—resolved. The aim of re-establishing the social status quo by first identifying then eliminating liminality is highlighted again by Kessler: "For the surgeon, the ambiguity signals an opportunity to fashion the inappropriate into the appropriate. Once the intersex marker has been corrected, the intersexed person (as intersexed) fades into the culture."[59] Once the liminal nature of the social actor is resolved, social discomfort ceases, since the person becomes socially unremarkable as simply another man or woman, boy or girl.

Though Turner writes about liminality as the mid-point in a rite of passage, many of the hallmark liminal attributes he identifies are relevant to the present discussion and include: transition (as noted above), anonymity, absence of status, total obedience, silence, suspension of rights, acceptance of pain and suffering, and heteronomy.[60] Because surgeons cannot inform intersexed children about surgeries when they are infants and, more importantly, because they often lie to the children when they are old enough to understand, the child's position is one of total obedience to medical authority (forced, rather than willed obedience), suspension of rights, and heteronomy. As Angela Moreno puts it, referring to the genital surgery to which she was subjected at age 12, "They didn't mention the part where they were going to slice off my clitoris. All of it. I guess the doctors assumed I was as horrified by my outsized clit as they were, and there was no need to discuss it with me."[61] And, as Morgan Holmes similarly writes, "Nobody asked me how I felt. . . . And they certainly didn't tell me they were going to amputate my clitoris."[62] Intersexual narratives such as these abound with claims of having been lied to and operated on at an age that is standardly acknowledged to mandate, at the very least, the assent of the child.[63] To deny a right as basic as the truth suggests that the intersexed child is somehow thought to fall outside the class of persons to whom such duties are owed: boys and girls, men and women, the unambiguous social actors of everyday structured life.

Insofar as these children and young adults seem not to have any choice in their treatment, they are expected, as are Turner's liminal persons, to obey and accept the pain and suffering associated with genital surgery.[64] As part of such forced acceptance, intersexuals frequently write about the silence and secrecy surrounding their condition as having made them voiceless, though it is a voicelessness now slowly being overcome. Many intersexuals (including several in this volume) write about never having been told their diagnosis, only to discover it alone, reading a medical textbook in a library after having heard, by chance, about modern day hermaphrodites. Others yet write about the secrecy surrounding their many surgeries and of never being able to talk about their condition with anyone else—friends or family—well into their adult years.[65] As Heidi Walcutt remarks, "We are all around you, but—until now—we have been *invisible* because we have been *silent.*"[66] Much like the liminal person without status—in other words, the person who is made structurally invisible—so too are many intersexuals rendered silent because the social categories available for others are unavailable for them. When one cannot be clearly identified, one should not be heard from.

Nor, for that matter, should one be spoken about. The invisibility and anonymity associated with liminal persons is also made manifest in the advice commonly given by physicians to parents of newborn intersexed children. In the first days after birth, physicians are trying to discover the cause of the intersexed condition and to determine which sex assignment (male or female) should be made for the intersexed child. In this liminal phase, physicians often recommend that parents refrain from naming the child and, indeed, from telling others the sex of the child. Rather, parents are asked to refer to the child neutrally as "the baby." Turner's remarks about liminal persons in a rite of passage are instructive here: liminal persons "have physical but not social 'reality,' hence they have to be hidden, since it is a paradox, a scandal, to see what ought not to be there!"[67] namely, "ambiguity" in something so fundamental as sex. Similarly, a story (perhaps apocryphal) is recounted of a couple whose child was born intersexed but who told everyone that they had newborn twins, one of each sex. Once the sex assignment had been made, the parents told friends that one of the twins had died.[68] The intersexed child is rendered invisible by being read metaphorically into the bodies of the twins, only later to be read out of existence, the liminality resolved.

Reconceiving of the medical management of intersexed children by focusing on Turner's notion of liminality accomplishes three things. First, it offers an alternate perspective on intersexuality that moves us away from the dysfunction model that underpins the medical viewpoint. Prior to invoking the work of Turner, I suggested that medical professionals pathologize the intersex condition by considering it to be a deviance or dysfunction in need of medical redress. By using the concept of liminality, the focus shifts from the idea of a pathology inherent in the intersexed body to a more explicitly socio-cultural account of the reasons for the current intersexual management philosophy: namely, that intersexed genitals, though strictly speaking not diseased, nonetheless challenge the validity of prevailing cultural categories and are thus felt to necessitate a surgical response. On this reading, the surgeon sculpts the genitals of the intersexed person, not because there is a medical dysfunction (for, in most cases, there clearly is not), but rather because the physician cannot fit the intersexed child into one of two available sex and gender categories. Second, the use of the notion of liminality further shows that our views about "ambiguity" are socially constructed and, therefore, open to criticism and revision. Through such criticism and revision, healthcare professionals may more easily begin "to see themselves not only as constrained by real world demands but as creators of that world,"[69] and, *following the lead of intersexuals themselves,* as agents of positive clinical and cultural change.

Finally, using liminality helps to frame the subjective experiences of intersexuals as recounted by intersexuals themselves. The experience of intersexed persons at the hands of surgeons appears to be uniformly negative.[70] Through the lens of liminality, the early experiences of intersexed persons are brought to expression and serve to strengthen the case for conceiving of intersexed persons as socially liminal. Most importantly, however, invoking the liminality framework opens up a social space for intersexed persons to reclaim authorship of their life stories and to create themselves anew as healthy, happy people. In this sense, liminality can serve to liberate intersexed persons from prevailing social structures because they themselves question the validity of the prevailing two-sex social structure and bring to light the fact that one can be an *intersexed* man or woman (rather than a *male-* or *female-sexed* man or woman) and be happy *as such.* While surgeons strive to move intersexed children out of their "ambiguous" state and into a male- or female-sexed state via surgery, intersexed persons voice a different, non-surgical emergence from liminality and, in so doing, eschew the prevalent two-sex worldview.

CONCLUSION

If the reasons behind the present treatment regimes for intersexuals are indeed cultural, then one way to alter our perceptions about our own practices is to look elsewhere and compare. As Elliott, on advice from Wittgenstein, suggests, one need only imagine that certain facts about our world are different in order for once-alien concepts to take on a familiar glow.[71] Similarly, as George Marcus and Michael Fischer suggest, "The juxtaposing of alien customs to familiar ones, or the relativizing of taken-for-granted concepts such as the family, power, and the beliefs that lend certainty to our everyday life, has the effect of disorienting the reader and altering perception."[72] Though many ideals have deep purchase with those within a culture, this need not mean that they are unshakable. In ways that are unclear, concepts and beliefs about the world can change, if imperceptibly at first, leaving people in a very different position than the one from which they started out. While the manner in which new concepts or ideas occupy and change the contours of cultural space remains unclear, what is certain is that a change of viewpoint is initially required. To effect change in thought, in other words, one must first be disoriented and look at things through different eyes.

For example, many non-Western societies have socially available (institutionalized) third sex/third gender categories, where the differently sexed person has a special (or, at least, acceptable) social gender role to play. In this context, one thinks of the Native American *berdaches*—males occupying female gender roles—who often take on a sacred role within the society; the *hijras* of India—emasculated males, some of whom undergo ritual castration—who can occupy either a male or a female gender role; and, finally, the *xaniths* of Oman—effeminate males—whose gender is more woman than man, but who retain their social status as males.[73] A recitation of such anthropological curios can have limited effect on the sceptic because we run up against a simple fact: we have the culture and society that we have, and while it is interesting to know that others conceive of things in different ways, the pathologizing of intersexuality that occurs in the West is a sad social fact that is *ours* to deal with.

This is a reasonable response, but these cases do nonetheless illustrate two basic points: first, they highlight the way in which a society *can* create social space for its actors by having in place sex and gender categories for those who are neither man nor woman, masculine nor feminine. Moreover, these examples act as counterpoints to our own social realities and can by juxtaposition prompt questions about our basic assumptions regarding the world. Put differently, if there are other places in the world where, say, third gender categories exist, or where intersexed persons can occupy a legitimate social role, then we may more easily see that part of the reaction to intersexed children is due to myopia-inducing cultural lenses. This is not to say that we can or should, as if by philosophical fiat, create a new sex or gender category to spread out over our social world. Rather, it is simply to say that our ideas about intersexuality are just that—ideas—and thus open to scrutiny and revision.

Yet another way to effect change in thought—one that I have attempted—is to remain within our own borders and to subject our practices and categories to scrutiny from within. The task here, as I have suggested, is also to look at the world through different eyes, namely, those of intersexed persons. In medical practice, there is a sometimes unfortunate tendency to, as it were, believe the body too much. In other words, if some feature that is not the norm expresses itself on or in the body, then a common reaction tends to be that this is a bad thing that needs to be eliminated. Often, perhaps most often, this is the correct response; often, however, it is not, as in the reaction to the variable genitals of intersexed children. The long-term impact of sex assignment surgeries on the gender identities of intersexed children is not dissimilar to the impact of cochlear implant surgery on the identities of prelingually deaf children. Though at first glance the deafness of a child may seem like an archetypal instance of a pathology in need of medical management, the full story is more complicated. For those deaf persons who use American Sign Language (ASL) and who identify with the Deaf community, to be Deaf is to be a member of an active cultural and linguistic minority group, rather than to be disabled.[74] Thought of in this way, and given the generally unimpressive results of cochlear implant surgery in helping many prelingually deaf children assimilate into the wider hearing society, arguments have been advanced in support of foregoing cochlear implant surgery in order to open up the possibility of the child becoming a member of the Deaf community.[75]

As with the case of prelingually deaf children, I have also argued that the reaction to the intersexed child is a cultural product of believing the body too much and, in particular, of "taking genitals too seriously."[76] Intersexed persons will be well-served if physicians follow Kessler's advice and start to take genitals less seriously, and to recognize that healthy and acceptable genitals can be highly variable without being "ambiguous" or "pathological." In a passage that starts off on a promising note, one suggesting the relative importance of gender over sex (and hence, by implication, over genital appearance), the intersex clinician New claims that "Society sees phenotype, not genotype," only to err by listing the genitals as among the phenotypic traits that society sees.[77] One need not embrace a postmodern version of the motto *in hoc signo vinces*[78]—that "gender is performance"—to realize that most of us who interact with the world and are recognized as being of one gender or the other do so without showing our genitals. As Kessler notes, the "fact that appearance is so important for a body part that is almost always hidden . . . is further evidence that more is at stake here than the body part itself."[79] What is at stake, as I've tried to show, is our (at times) unreflective acceptance of existing socio-cultural categories, as well as the medical profession's insistence on the deterministic relation between genital appearance and gender role. The intersexed child can be assigned as a boy or a girl *without requiring any genital surgery at all*. Should they so choose, intersexed men and women can have the optional genital surgery later when they are old enough to decide for themselves.

Mary Douglas, writing over 30 years ago, noted that there "are several ways of treating anomalies. Negatively, we can ignore, just not perceive them, or perceiving we can condemn. Positively we can deliberately confront the anomaly and try to create a new pattern of reality in which it has a place."[80] Similarly, Turner writes, "Either you can say, like the little boy on first seeing a giraffe, 'I don't believe it,' and deny the social existence of the biological fact; or else, having accepted the fact, you can try to cope with it."[81] I suggest that we, as Douglas and Turner long ago suggested, adopt the second strategy in our approach to intersexed children. As I suggested at the outset, the problem with "ambiguity" and with intersexed persons is really a problem with the rest of us and, thus, it is up to the rest of us to rethink our views.

As evidenced by the Deaf community/cochlear implant debate, great advances in understanding can be made when a condition is depathologized and people stop to listen to those who are subject to the medical technologies that are brought to bear on the assumed pathology. It is, after all, those who are subject to such technologies whose lives are affected. The fact remains that the current management philosophy is arguably a failure and has clearly produced a large number of unhappy people.[82] As William Reiner has rightly claimed, "it is only the children themselves who can and must identify who and what they are. It is for us as clinicians and researchers to listen and to learn."[83] By overcoming the urge to try to make real persons conform to ideal forms—and, thus, in decoupling genitals from gender—it will become clear that it is well within the realm of possibility that intersexed women with larger than typical clitorises and small or absent vaginas can lead healthy, fulfilling lives and be happy; so too is it possible that intersexed men with smaller than typical penises can lead healthy, fulfilling lives and be happy.[84] Presumably, medical professionals have the best interests and the happiness of their patients as their ultimate goal; they need only open their minds to the perspective of patients, past and present, and take Holmes' advice: "Please listen to us as we tell you how to meet that goal."[85]

ACKNOWLEDGMENTS

I would like to thank Liam Buckley, Carl Elliott, Barb Secker, Shelly Skinner, Edie Turner, and Anna Zalewski for very thoughtful comments on previous drafts of this article. I am grateful to Suzanne Kessler for permission to cite from her book, *Lessons from the Intersexed.* For permission to cite from her work, I thank Kiira Triea. Finally, I owe Alice Dreger an especially large debt for initially involving me in this project and for giving me outstanding assistance throughout.

This chapter first appeared in *The Journal of Clinical Ethics* 9, no. 4 (Winter 1998); © 1998 by *The Journal of Clinical Ethics*; used with permission.

NOTES

1. J. Lorber, *Paradoxes of Gender* (New Haven, Conn.: Yale University Press, 1994), 13.

2. T. Laqueur, *Making Sex: Body and Gender from the Greeks to Freud* (Cambridge, Mass.: Harvard University Press, 1990), 135.

3. S.J. Kessler, *Lessons from the Intersexed* (New Brunswick, N.J.: Rutgers University Press, 1998), 5.

4. J. Diamond, "Turning a Man," *Discover* 13 (1992): 70-77, 77.

5. Lorber, *Paradoxes of Gender*, see note 1 above, p. 14; emphasis added.

6. L.A. Parker, "Ambiguous Genitalia: Etiology, Treatment, and Nursing Implications," *Journal of Obstetric, Gynecologic, & Neonatal Nursing* 27 (1998): 15-22, 15.

7. G. Izquierdo and K.I. Glassberg, "Gender Assignment and Gender Identity in Patients with Ambiguous Genitalia," *Urology* 42 (1993): 232-42, 232.

8. S.A. Taha, "Male Pseudohermaphroditism: Factors Determining the Gender of Rearing in Saudi Arabia," *Urology* 43 (1994): 370-74, 370.

9. C.H. Meyers-Seifer and N.J. Charest, "Diagnosis and Management of Patients with Ambiguous Genitalia," *Seminars in Perinatology* 16 (1992): 332-39, 332.

10. M.I. New, "Female Pseudohermaphroditism," *Seminars in Perinatology* 16 (1992): 299-318, 311.

11. For example, medical treatment is required when intersexed children are diagnosed with the salt-wasting form of congenital adrenal hyperplasia (CAH), a potentially fatal variety of the endocrine condition that causes virilization (masculinization) of the external genitalia in females (e.g., larger than statistically normal clitoris), but which is harder to detect in males. See ibid. The importance of prompt medical treatment when necessary is clearly endorsed by A.D. Dreger, " 'Ambiguous Sex'—or Ambivalent Medicine? Ethical Issues in the Treatment of Intersexuality," *Hastings Center Report* 28 (1998): 24-35, 30.

12. A.D. Dreger, *Hermaphrodites and the Medical Invention of Sex* (Cambridge, Mass.: Harvard University Press, 1998), especially chapter 5.

13. A. Fausto-Sterling, "How to Build a Man," in *Science and Homosexualities*, ed. V.A. Rosario (New York: Routledge, 1997), 219-25.

14. J. Money, J.G. Hampson, and J.L. Hampson, "Hermaphroditism: Recommendations Concerning Assignment of Sex, Change of Sex, and Psychological Management," *Bulletin of the Johns Hopkins Hospital* 97 (1955): 284-300; ibid., "An Examination of Some Basic Sexual Concepts: The Evidence of Human

Hermaphroditism," *Bulletin of the Johns Hopkins Hospital* 97 (1955): 301-19; and ibid., "Imprinting and the Establishment of Gender Role," *Archives of Neurology and Psychiatry* 79 (1957): 333-37.

15. For a critique, see M. Diamond, "Sexual Identity and Sexual Orientation in Children with Traumatized or Ambiguous Genitalia," *Journal of Sex Research* 34 (1997): 199-211.

16. Dreger, " 'Ambiguous Sex', " see note 11 above, pp. 27-29.

17. P.K. Donahue, "The Diagnosis and Treatment of Infants with Intersex Abnormalities," *Pediatric Clinics of North America* 34 (1987): 1333-48. "Clitoris" and "vagina" are placed in quotes here because a clitoris or vagina on a surgically assigned male pseudohermaphrodite refer to something very different than a clitoris or vagina on the average woman—in the former case, they are a clitoris and vagina in appearance only; in the latter, a clitoris and vagina in appearance and sexual responsiveness. The same comments hold true for surgically constructed labia.

18. J.W. Duckett and L.S. Baskin, "Genitoplasty for Intersex Anomalies," *European Journal of Pediatrics* 152, suppl. 2 (1993): S80-S84, S83.

19. New, "Female Pseudohermaphroditism," see note 10 above, p. 311.

20. W.G. Reiner, "Sex Assignment in the Neonate With Intersex or Inadequate Genitalia," *Archives of Pediatric and Adolescent Medicine* 151 (1997): 1044-45; and ibid., "To Be Male or Female—That Is the Question," *Archives of Pediatric and Adolescent Medicine* 151 (1997): 224-25.

21. Z. Krstic et al., "Surgical Treatment of Intersex Disorders," *Journal of Pediatric Surgery* 30 (1995): 1273-81, 1277.

22. Kessler, *Lessons from the Intersexed,* see note 3 above, p. 39.

23. Various writers, as quoted in ibid., pp. 35-36.

24. Surgeons, of course, have been trying new techniques in order to preserve clitoral sensation, but often adopt highly reductive measures to estimate the remaining sexual sensation. For one such attempt, and a brief critique, see, respectively: J.P. Gearhart et al., "Measurement of Pudental Evoked Potentials During Feminizing Genitoplasty: Technique and Applications," *Journal of Urology* 153 (1995): 486-87; and C. Chase, "Letters to the Editor, RE: Measurement of Pudental Evoked Potentials During Feminizing Genitoplasty: Technique and Applications," *Journal of Urology* 156 (1996): 1139-40. The point is simply that neural activity may be a poor estimator of sexual phenomenology.

25. Krstic et al., "Surgical Treatment," see note 21 above, p. 1280.

26. As quoted in Kessler, *Lessons from the Intersexed,* see note 3 above, p. 57.

27. There may well be cognitive traces from *in utero* exposures to hormones that affect gender role later during childhood. Exactly how powerful these early hormonal influences are in determining later gender identity is a debated issue, but all agree that such hormonal exposures do have a significant role to play. For two case studies that have different outcomes, see: M. Diamond and K. Sigmundson, "Sex Reassignment at Birth: Long-term Review and Clinical Implications," *Archives of Pediatric and Adolescent Medicine* 151 (1997):

298-304; and, S.J. Bradley et al., "Experiment in Nurture: Ablatio Penis at 2 Months, Sex Reassignment at 7 Months, and a Psychosexual Follow-up in Young Adulthood," *Pediatrics* 102 (1998): e9 (full text is available only on-line: < http:///www.pediatrics.org/cgi/contents/full/102/1/e9 >. More generally, see: M. Diamond et al., "From Fertilization to Adult Sexual Behavior," *Hormones and Behavior* 30 (1996): 333-53.

28. As quoted in Kessler, *Lessons from the Intersexed,* see note 3 above, p. 37.

29. A.P. van Seters and A.K. Slob, "Mutually Gratifying Heterosexual Relationship with Micropenis of Husband," *Journal of Sex & Marital Therapy* 14 (1988): 98-107; and, J.M. Reilly and C.R.J. Woodhouse, "Small Penis and the Male Sexual Role," *Journal of Urology* 142 (1989): 569-71.

30. J. Fichtner, "Analysis of Meatal Location in 500 Men: Wide Variation Questions Need for Meatal Advancement in All Pediatric Anterior Hypospadias Cases," *Journal of Urology* 154 (1995): 833-34.

31. As quoted in Kessler, *Lessons from the Intersexed,* see note 3 above, p. 70.

32. As Kessler notes, in the latter case the "male's *manliness* might be at stake," while in the former case "his essential *maleness* might be." Ibid., p. 19.

33. Fausto-Sterling, "How to Build a Man," see note 13 above, p. 222.

34. This is perhaps most apparent in certain Muslim societies where male pseudohermaphrodites with micropenis almost universally choose to remain in the masculine gender role because the society in which they live is so patriarchal that men enjoy much greater financial and social benefits than women. See H.M. Al-Attia, "Gender Identity and Role in a Pedigree of Arabs with Intersex due to 5 Alpha Reductase-2 Deficiency," *Psychoneuroendocrinology* 21 (1996): 651-57; A. Farkas and A. Rosler, "Ten Years Experience with Masculinizing Genitoplasty in Male Pseudohermaphroditism due to 17b-Hydroxysteroid Dehydrogenase Deficiency," *European Journal of Pediatrics* 152, suppl. 2 (1993): S88-S90; and Taha, "Male Pseudohermaphroditism," see note 8 above.

35. Lorber, *Paradoxes of Gender,* see note 1 above, p. 22. On gender ascription, see S.J. Kessler and W. McKenna, *Gender: An Ethnomethodological Approach* (Chicago: University of Chicago Press, 1978).

36. One shocking example of gender ascription occurring when the child is rewarded for "gender-appropriate" behavior is the story of the parent who noticed that different awards were being given out to the boys and girls in her son's kindergarten classroom. The boys were given Very Best Thinker, Most Eager Learner, Most Imaginative, Mr. Personality, and Hardest Worker awards; while the girls were given All-Around Sweetheart, Sweetest Personality, Cutest Personality, Best Manners, and Best Helper awards. This story is recounted in D.L. Rhode, *Speaking of Sex: The Denial of Gender Inequality* (Cambridge, Mass.: Harvard University Press, 1997), 55.

37. Unfortunately, part of the story concerning the treatment of intersexed persons involves an implicit heterosexism, or perhaps more accurately, an implicit homophobia on the part of medical professionals. As New puts it " . . . one of the major goals of therapy is to ensure that gender role, gender behavior,

and gender identity are isosexual with the sex of assignment." In other words, sexual orientation is read into sex and gender, such that to be male means to be attracted to women, while to be female means to be attracted to men. New, "Female Pseudohermaphroditism," see note 10 above, p. 311.

38. K. Triea, "Finishing School Dropout," < http://www.qis.net/~triea/ finish.html > (1996).

39. Lorber considers such practices as binding the feet of Chinese girls, circumcising the penises of Jewish boys, and surgically augmenting the breasts of women to be examples of gender inscription on the body. Lorber, *Paradoxes of Gender*, see note 1 above, p. 24.

40. C. Elliott, "Can't We Go On As Three?" *Hastings Center Report* 28 (1998): 36-39, 39.

41. Kessler, *Lessons from the Intersexed*, see note 3 above, p. 75.

42. Diamond, "Turning a Man," see note 4 above, p. 72.

43. Ibid., 77.

44. Kessler, *Lessons from the Intersexed*, see note 3 above, p. 8.

45. Ibid., p. 118; emphasis added.

46. Lorber, *Paradoxes of Gender*, see note 1 above, pp. 32-35.

47. Rhode, *Speaking of Sex*, see note 36 above.

48. My claim here is not that all structures, or social categories, are universal across cultures and thus function in the same way. My point is simply that in many cross-cultural comparisons, certain categories will structure social relations is similar ways. For an interesting discussion of where this is not true, see M. Strathern, "No Nature, No Culture: The Hagen Case," in *Nature, Culture and Gender*, ed. C. MacCormack, and M. Strathern (London: Cambridge University Press, 1980): 174-222.

49. V.W. Turner, *Dramas, Fields, and Metaphors: Symbolic Action in Human Society* (Ithaca, N.Y.: Cornell University Press, 1974), 237.

50. V.W. Turner, *The Ritual Process: Structure and Anti-Structure* (Harmondsworth, England: Penguin Books Ltd., 1969), 114-15.

51. Turner, *Dramas, Fields, and Metaphors*, see note 49 above, p. 237.

52. Turner, *The Ritual Process*, see note 50 above, p. 112.

53. Turner's interest here is in rites of passage in traditional societies where people pass from a role and status position (structure), through an undifferentiated, role- and status-less liminal state (anti-structure), and on to a new role and status position (structure). My focus is on the liminal phase, extracted from the process of ritual.

54. Turner, *The Ritual Process*, see note 50 above, p. 81.

55. V.W. Turner, *The Forest of Symbols: Aspects of Ndembu Ritual* (Ithaca, N.Y.: Cornell University Press, 1967), p. 96.

56. Turner, *Dramas, Fields, and Metaphors*, see note 49 above, p. 268.

57. Turner, *The Forest of Symbols*, see note 55 above, p. 95.

58. Kessler, *Lessons from the Intersexed*, see note 3 above, p. 31.

59. Ibid., p. 5.

60. Turner, *The Ritual Process,* see note 50 above, pp. 92-93.

61. A. Moreno, "In Amerika They Call Us Hermaphrodites," chapter 13 of this volume.

62. M. Holmes, "Is Growing Up in Silence Better Than Growing Up Different?" *Chrysalis: The Journal of Transgressive Gender Identities* 2 (1997/1998): 7-9, 8.

63. Committee on Bioethics, "Informed Consent, Parental Permission, and Assent in Pediatric Practice," *Pediatrics* 95 (1995): 314-17.

64. Kessler notes how some of the follow-up treatment for gender-assigned females, as well as the excessive number of genital exams, is *felt* by parents (as well, one presumes, by children) as a form of abuse. Kessler, *Lessons from the Intersexed,* see note 3 above, pp. 59, 63. John Money and Margaret Lamacz also note how genital examinations can be experienced subjectively by children as a form of sexual abuse. The authors suggest caution when performing such exams, "even if only for self-protection." In a passage that is nothing short of offensive, they conclude, making the self-serving nature of the article apparent: "Streetwise children have already learned their power of vengeance by falsely accusing an adult of sexual abuse, and their parents have learned how much malpractice or divorce money it can be worth. . . . Do not forget that, in the victimology industry, the official sexual abuse doctrine is that children never lie." J. Money and M. Lamacz, "Genital Examination and Exposure Experienced as Nosocomial Sexual Abuse in Childhood," *Journal of Nervous and Mental Disease* 175 (1987): 713-21, 720-21.

65. On the silence and secrecy experienced by intersexed persons see [Anonymous], "Once a Dark Secret," *British Medical Journal* 308 (1994): 542; and various writers in the "Intersex Awakening" issue of *Chrysalis: The Journal of Transgressive Gender Identities* 2 (1997/1998): 1-56. Further intersex sources are to be found on the Intersex Society of North America (ISNA) website, < http://www.isna.org >, and on the Intersex Voices website, < http://www.qis.net/ ~triea >.

66. H. Walcutt, "Time For a Change," chapter 19 of this volume.

67. Turner, *The Forest of Symbols,* see note 55 above, p. 98.

68. This story is told in Kessler, *Lessons from the Intersexed,* see note 3 above, p. 21.

69. Ibid., p. 120.

70. Of course, there are intersexed persons who have not come forward to tell their stories, and one is thus left to ponder whether some of these people have had better experiences with the medical "treatments" they received.

71. Elliott, "Can't We Go On As Three?" see note 40 above, p. 36.

72. G.E. Marcus and M.M.J. Fischer, *Anthropology as Cultural Critique: An Experimental Moment in the Human Sciences* (Chicago: University of Chicago Press, 1986), 111.

73. On these, see the brief discussion in Lorber, *Paradoxes of Gender,* see note 1 above, pp. 90-95. On the *berdache,* see W. Roscoe, "How to Become a

Berdache: Toward a Unified Analysis of Gender Diversity," in *Third Sex, Third Gender: Beyond Sexual Dimorphism in Culture and History,* ed. G. Herdt (New York: Zone Books, 1996): 329-72; and on the hijras, see S. Nanda, "Hijras: An Alternative Sex and Gender Role in India," ibid., pp. 373-417.

74. C. Padden and T. Humphreys, *Deaf in America: Voices from a Culture* (Cambridge, Mass.: Harvard University Press, 1989).

75. H. Lane and M. Grodin, "Ethical Issues in Cochlear Implant Surgery: An Exploration into Disease, Disability, and the Best Interests of the Child," *Kennedy Institute of Ethics Journal* 7 (1997): 231-51; and, R.A. Crouch, "Letting the deaf Be Deaf: Reconsidering the Use of Cochlear Implants in Prelingually Deaf Children," *Hastings Center Report* 27 (1997): 14-21.

76. Kessler, *Lessons from the Intersexed,* see note 3 above, p. 90.

77. New, "Female Pseudohermaphroditism," see note 10 above, p. 311.

78. ["In this sign thou shalt conquer." According to legend, the Emperor Constantine saw these words on a cross before an important battle, and converted to Christianity on his victory.—ED.]

79. Kessler, *Lessons from the Intersexed,* see note 3 above, p. 126.

80. M. Douglas, *Purity and Danger: An Analysis of Concepts of Pollution and Taboo* (London: Routledge & Kegan Paul, 1966), 38.

81. Turner, *The Ritual Process,* see note 50 above, p. 45.

82. Dreger, " 'Ambiguous Sex' " see note 11 above.

83. Reiner, "To Be Male or Female," see note 20 above, p. 225.

84. Diamond, "Sexual Identity and Sexual Orientation," see note 15 above; and Reilly and Woodhouse, "Small Penis and the Male Sexual Role," see note 29 above.

85. M. Holmes, "Is Growing Up in Silence," see note 62 above, p. 9.

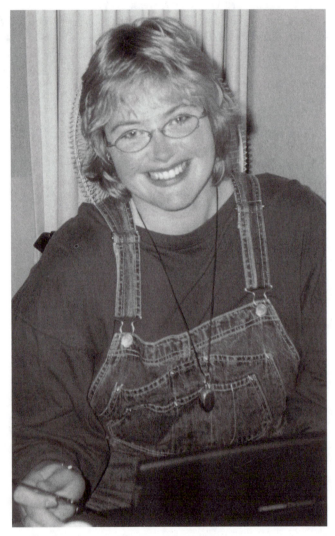

Sharon E. Preves

4

For the Sake of the Children: Destigmatizing Intersexuality

Sharon E. Preves

> It's as though you take a child who's born with Down's syndrome and has a certain appearance and you do cosmetic surgery to make them look like everyone else; you say, "They don't look different; they're not different." . . .
> You're not going to admit that they're different because the whole point of changing them is so that they're not different anymore and now the problem is fixed, erased . . . and what a disaster that is. If they didn't have some special help and they needed it. But the whole point is that you've erased the problem. You don't have to do anything.
> —Excerpt from the author's interview with "Joseph"

This article explores the process by which contemporary North American medicine attempts to "normalize" individuals who are born intersexed. The particular medical aims to normalize intersexuals and their families have been articulated in this book and elsewhere. The purpose of my contribution is to impart the experience of such interventions as told by intersexuals themselves. I provide a preliminary report on intersexuals' experiences as conveyed to me during in-depth life history interviews with 41 adults born sexually ambiguous.[1] I found that medical attempts aimed at destigmatizing intersexuality are experienced as alienating and shaming. I also found that many intersexuals are engaged in reclaiming intersexuality as a positive and empowering aspect of self.

The sexing of babies at birth as either female or male is one of the most rudimentary demarcations of North American culture. Once an infant's sex is ascertained, sex-appropriate gender socialization may begin. When an infant is not "sexable" because of genital or other anatomical obscurity, its entrance into the social world may be halted until the child is sexed. Because sex and gender provide expectations for a majority of our social interactions, the inability to sex an individual is extremely problematic socially. Clarity of sex grants an individual "personhood";[2] an ability to be considered human rather than monster or sub-human.[3] Despite the typically medically benign occurrence of intersexuality,[4] the social problem of sexlessness and the medicalization of childbirth lead to the social definition of the intersexed body as a diseased body. Due to a limited understanding of sex and gender, reinforced by a strongly gender-dichotomous and heteronormative culture,[5] intersexed individuals have been characterized as abnormal and in need of medical intervention to spare them from becoming social and sexual "freaks."[6]

The case of an intersex birth, a birth at which one's sex cannot readily be ascertained, announced, and counted upon, provides a poignant example of normative expectations remaining unfulfilled. According to sociologist Harold Garfinkel,[7] we are able to ascertain the strength and specific nature of social norms by deviating from them and closely gauging the response. This method, known as ethnomethodology, stems from an understanding of the three basic elements of social deviance. These elements are (1) the existence of a shared social expectation; (2) a marked violation or deviation from the prevailing social expectation; and (3) the social response to such a deviation. Gauging the social response to normative violations is key to understanding the salience of the initial social expectation.

In applying this model to intersex, the social expectation is that babies are born as one of two clearly delineated anatomical types—female or male—as ascertained by genital presentation at birth. In the case of intersexuality, normative violation occurs when genitalia and/or later pubescent development are not congruent with a two-sex model. North American social reaction to this form of deviance is primarily medical, due to the medicalization of childbirth and the medicalization of normality in this culture. The specific response to intersexual "deviance" is so strong that we have developed institutional means of covering up or erasing the violation, so that the initial social expectation of sex binarism may be upheld. More specifically, we have created medical means of surgically and hormonally engineering bodies that adhere to a two-sex social system.

Why would a cultural institution go to such great lengths to uphold a two-sex system when there are clearly consistent exceptions to this norm? One reason is that, because intersex is incongruent with the predominant, binary understanding of sex and gender, it generates the potential for social stigma and identity confusion.[8] According to sociologist Erving Goffman, stigma connotes a quality of immorality and inhumanity about the bearer of the imperfection, and prevents a person or group from achieving total social acceptance. In the 1950s, U.S. clinicians developed recommendations for surgical and hormonal sex assignment to preclude such trauma.[9]

The work of psychologist John Money is at the center of late 20th century debates on how to respond to intersexuality. Money's and others' research in this area emphasizes the psychological need to medically clarify the sex of intersexed infants at birth to alleviate the social stigma that could potentially arise from sexual ambiguity.[10] At the center of this treatment model is the objective of normative psychosocial development of intersexed children as clearly sexed individuals. It is precisely "for the sake of the children" (and their families)—in the hope of preventing social isolation and stigma—that cosmetic and other alterations of intersexed bodies are performed. In this case, "for the sake of the child" requires erasure of difference. More specifically, according to this model, sexual ambiguity must be eradicated or hidden from view in order for intersexuals and their families to be granted normative social space.

A need for discretion regarding an intersexual's true physical state is quite sensible if one subscribes to the prevailing treatment model, whose primary concern is "optimal gender" outcome, where clear gender identity is the objective.[11] One of the main tenets of the optimal gender theory is to prevent any overt attention to an intersexed child's anatomical difference. According to this model, optimal gender outcome is attainable only if an intersexed child receives congruent and consistent messages about her/his sexual anatomy and (presumed) gender throughout childhood. In order to assure parents' ability to uphold sex/gender clarity for their child, the family of an intersexed child must also receive information that reinforces their ability to uphold the "true sex" of that child. Unfortunately, this focus on gender clarity may lead to parents and/or children receiving misinformation or incomplete information about an intersexual's actual physical makeup.[12]

Despite the medical aim to abolish the stigmatized intersexed category, some intersexuals are finding each other through their own activism and are attempting to reclaim portions of their stigmatized identities as empowering and freeing.[13] In addition, some scholars and adult intersexuals are questioning the ethics and effectiveness of contemporary North American medical intervention on intersexed children.[14]

As a means of understanding the burgeoning intersex social movement and criticism geared at contemporary North American medical intervention, I set out to explore how these attempts at destigmatization are experienced by intersexuals.

METHODS

Between May of 1997 and September of 1998 I conducted 41 in-depth, life history interviews with adults who were born intersexed.[15] Participants range in age from 20 to 65, with a mean age of 40. The participants live throughout North America and are predominantly, but not entirely, Caucasian, middle-class, and college educated. The majority of interviews took place in the participants' homes. I initially recruited participants from a variety of intersex support groups, including the Androgen Insensitivity Support Group U.S.; the Androgen Insensitivity Support Group of Canada; the Coalition for Intersex Support, Activism, and Education; the Congenital Adrenal Hyperplasia Network; the Hermaphrodite Education and Listening Post; the Intersex Society of Canada; the Intersex Society of North America; the Intersex Support Group International; and the Middlesex Group. I conducted additional recruitment through social network sampling, that is, referrals from initial research participants.

The interviews concentrate on participants' life histories with specific attention to how they learned of their intersexuality, experiences with medical intervention, issues of identity development, and significance of social support. In addition, the interviews explore participants' sexual identities, their experience of gender and sexual identity development, challenges associated with being intersexed, and how they respond to those challenges. The interviews are approximately two and one-half hours in length, are tape recorded, and transcribed. Using a qualitative computer data analysis program (ATLAS/ti), I closely analyze interview and field note data for thematic patterns in content.[16]

The members of the social support and advocacy organizations from which I sampled cannot be expected to represent the diversity of experience within the intersex population. In fact, because there has been so little clinical follow up on intersexuals, I don't presume to know what the constitution of that population actually is. Rather, these organizations serve as a strategic and theoretically promising sampling base, given the social context of an emerging intersex social movement.

It is important to note that there is significant diversity within and among the existing 16 North American intersex support, advocacy, and education organizations. Unlike some who view the members of these organizations as a cohesive community represented best by the Intersex Society of North America (ISNA)—which has been perhaps the most vocal of these advocacy groups[17]—I encountered a rich diversity of sexual identities and opinions about medical intervention on intersexed infants and children among the people I interviewed. In fact, several disassociated themselves from the category of "intersex," even though, diagnostically, their physiology would be so classified. Many individuals also seemed to participate in upholding a two-sex system by engaging in classically "feminine" or "masculine" behaviors and roles and participating in what would be outwardly perceived as heterosexual activity—that is, sexual activity with partners who were sexed "opposite." Among some of the more gender traditional participants, I encountered individuals who distanced themselves from the well-publicized lobbying efforts of certain intersex activists to stop "cosmetic" genital surgery on intersexuals, saying such things as, "You know I'm not part of that radical lobbying group, right?"

FINDINGS

The findings of this research extend far beyond what I have space to report in this article. The data on which I focus here are specific to intersexuals' experiences of medicalization and living with bodies that have been classified as deviant. I organize the data by first reporting on the experience of medicalization as shaming and then reporting on ways in which intersexuals have coped with being marginalized via models of "coming out" and community empowerment.

Despite the striking variation of identities and politics represented in the sample, I found amazing consistency among individuals' experiences with medical attempts to "normalize" their bodies. Throughout the interviews, individuals conveyed that being encouraged to keep silent about their differences and surgical alterations only served to enforce feelings of isolation, stigma, and shame—the very feelings that such procedures are attempting to alleviate. Individuals repeatedly raised issues of wanting autonomy over their bodies, longing to talk with others who had similar anatomy, and wanting to participate in decision making related to medical intervention. Of those who had recurring medical examinations or treatments to clarify sex assignment, I found the feelings of shame to be most intense. These individuals spoke of feeling "monstrous, Other, and freakish." In stark contrast, when the very same individuals spoke of gaining accurate information about their bodies, telling others openly about their physical differences, and finding other intersexuals with whom to relate, they related feelings of pride about their difference and their identities. It is important to note that although optimal gender theory aims to de-emphasize physical difference, medical practitioners pay significant attention to intersexuals' ambiguous anatomy during physical exams.

FEARING THE UNKNOWN:
"WHAT KIND OF MONSTER AM I?"

One of the most common themes I heard in intersexuals' stories centers around a lack of full disclosure on the part of clinicians and family members regarding the nature of intersexed conditions. For example, in speaking of the silence and secrecy she experienced in her late twenties when trying to ascertain the details of her own anatomy from her physicians, Sarah said, "And they wouldn't tell me anything. I knew that there was more to it than all this. . . . I knew that I wasn't being told the truth but there was no way anybody was gonna tell me the truth. It was such a mess. There was so much lying and symboling going on that there's a wonder I ever figured it out. . . . Most everybody's figured it out for themselves."

Greta, Max, and Claire each spoke about the impact of such a lack of disclosure. In Greta's words, "Because there was no information and it was withheld it was a huge issue, and it greatly affected my sense of self because I was constantly questioning who I was." According to Max, "Intersexuals aren't encouraged to be autonomous, period. I mean, who we are is dictated to us. That's been my experience. And that's why I had no identity and I struggled so hard to find one." And in Claire's words, "[There was] total and complete silence. You know, it was never, never mentioned. And, you know, I mean . . . I know you know what that does. And I was just in agony trying to figure out who I was. And you know, why . . . what sex I was. And feeling like a freak, which is a very common story. And then when I was 12 I asked my father what had been done to me. And his answer was, 'Don't be so self-examining.' And that was it. I never asked again [until I was 35]."

As in Sarah and Claire's cases, most participants shared histories of searching for information about their different bodies; about trying to piece the puzzle together for themselves. Many told of attempting to retrieve medical records and requesting information of their parents, to no avail. In their persistence and desperation to make sense of their medicalized histories, several began searching for information about themselves in medical texts at public or university libraries.

According to the participants, lacking information about their bodies and medical histories was far more difficult than actually knowing the truth. Several shared stories about imagining they had terminal illnesses or disorders too freakish to comprehend, let alone discuss. In Max's words, "What I knew myself to be was too horrible; I wasn't a viable fetus." In another case Flora had the following experience with a genetic counselor when she was 24: "[The geneticist] said . . . 'I'm obliged to tell you that certain details of your condition have not been divulged to you, but I cannot tell you what they are because they would upset you too much.' So she's telling us we don't know everything, but she can't tell us what it is because it's too horrible."

It is standard practice to sex individuals born with complete androgen insensitivity syndrome (CAIS) as female, as they lack the ability to masculinize due to an inability to respond to male hormones. These individuals are often not told that they possess both XY chromosomes and undescended testicles. Typically the testes of people with CAIS are removed via orchiectomy in adolescence, or earlier, due to the possibility that they could become cancerous. In keeping with the optimal gender theory, it is also standard to refer to the organs removed during this surgery generically as "gonads" or "precancerous ovaries" to downplay the discord between a female sex assignment and typically male anatomy. Concealing the fact that testes are actually the organs being removed during this operation has recently been considered medically ethical. (For example, in 1995, a medical student won second place in the Logie Medical Ethics Essay Contest of the *Canadian Medical Association Journal* for an essay that justified deception of AIS patients, including adults.)[18] On the experience of being lied to about having precancerous ovaries Ana said, "And then . . . the doctor started talking to me about my ovaries . . . she probably actually said, 'There's a great likelihood that you'll develop cancer very soon and we have to have your ovaries out immediately.' But all I heard was cancer. I . . . spent all my teenage years terrified I was gonna die someday riddled with cancer."

Having a similar experience with lack of complete disclosure during the removal of her undescended testicles, Greta also spoke of fearing that she would someday develop cancer or some other life-threatening illness. When she learned the truth about her surgery and about what caused her body to be different, Greta stated that not knowing the truth had been far more damaging than learning what had been withheld from her. In her own words, "I was devastated because . . . I sort of had an inkling of, 'Oh my God, there's something not right here.'. . . I finally had a label for [it] and I had to deal with the fact that it had been withheld from me . . . [and] THAT was the big secret? THAT was the big secret? You know, like, 'hello,' that's nothing. That's like nothing."

ERASING DIFFERENCE

In addition to experiencing the unknown as frightening and shaming, many who had genital surgeries emphasized that the very operations that were intended to assuage feelings of difference only served to highlight their stigma. In reflecting upon the clitoral recession she received at age seven, Faye said, "I looked back on it and thought, this must have been really necessary. And that sort of went with me through childhood. If they would do this to me, it must be that I'm unacceptable as I am. The point is the emotional damage you do by telling someone that 'You're so fucking ugly that we couldn't send you home to your parents the way you were.' I mean, give the parents some credit. Teach them. Help them to deal with their different child."

While it is common to perform surgery on the external genitalia of young children, internal operations such as vaginoplasty (the surgical creation of a vagina from skin or colon grafts) are sometimes not performed until the teen years. Although the surgery takes place later, messages about its impending necessity are common throughout childhood. In reference to conversation about vaginoplasty with a physician at age 15, Max said, "I had always been told that I was a girl, I just wasn't finished and I was going to need to have this surgery eventually . . . that this would be necessary because I was a girl but I wasn't finished and this is how they would finish me."

Commonly, manual vaginal dilation is used in conjuncture with vaginoplasty. Some intersexuals who are sexed as female do not undergo vaginoplasty, but may be encouraged to lengthen and widen their existing vaginal openings via manual dilation with a dildo. Many relayed embarrassing tales of pubescent conversations in doctors' offices (often times with parents present) where physicians were instructing them how to use medically produced dildos to increase the penetrative capacity of their vaginas. In her own words, Ana said, "At that time she told me I would need to [dilate] like two or three times a day for at least 20 minutes at a time—just like hold it there. And I'm living in a dorm, you know? It was pretty impossible. I found it so humiliating and just degrading that I think I didn't do it [even a total of] three times. I just couldn't, you know. I just couldn't do it. And I felt a little like a failure about that."

Despite the humiliation and disgrace communicated in each story, each one of the individuals I interviewed persisted in gaining accurate and complete information about their bodies and their histories. In addition, each person was determined to find others who were like her or him, convinced that others in fact did exist despite tales of the rarity of intersexuality.

MODELS OF COMING OUT AND COMMUNITY EMPOWERMENT

I have organized the data in this article as they appeared in the interviews. The first half of most interviews was laden with tales of pain, sorrow, bewilderment, and anger; the second half encompassed accounts of empowerment, identification, and reappropriation of intersexuality as a positive aspect of self. Through their association with various intersex support and/or advocacy organizations, all participants related narratives of coping with the stigma of difference through "coming out" rather than assimilating to the norm.

Several researchers have explored individuals' means of living with various stigmatized characteristics, such as physical disability. In their work in this area Anspach, Barnard, Hahn, Sudsman, and Yoshida detail the ways in which individuals gain pride in their stigmatized identities through political activism, autonomy, and visibility.[19] Related to activism, identifying with others who have been similarly outcast increases one's sense of efficacy in creating her/his own identity. Through this empowerment, individuals work to counteract Goffman's notion of a spoiled identity.[20] In the case of intersexuality, the recent development of more than one dozen support and advocacy groups provides an interesting opportunity to not only study the identity politics of a social movement, but to more clearly understand how some intersexuals may experience and respond to extant social expectations of sex and gender via coming out and community empowerment.

Models of coming out identify a multi-stage process of embracing one's identity. These stages include: (1) recognition of one's non-conformity; (2) acknowledgment of one's difference to self and others; (3) seeking and socializing with similar others; (4) pride in the marginal identity; and (5) integration of one's identity within a prevailing socio-cultural context.[21] Empirical investigation of how gays and lesbians cope with such stigma has contributed to an understanding of this coming-out process. Theorists and activists have subsequently applied the "coming-out" model to transgender individuals. Stone called for transgender people to come out and affirm their unique transsexual identities that transcend the heterosexual imperatives.[22] Bockting discussed the implications of coming out for the clinical management of gender dysphoria.[23] Similar to persons with disabilities, these groups seek empowerment and, by organizing themselves, transform a stigmatized identity into one of dignity and pride. Based on my research and the research of others, I would argue that we are currently witnessing a similar trend among intersex individuals.[24]

For example, on recognizing their difference—as in the first stage of coming out—Flora, Faye, and Mel each speak of this first stage of acknowledgment as a positive experience. In Flora's words, "So [the doctor] told me what it was and I was relieved. Not only was I relieved, but what I first felt about it was . . . I felt kinda special. I thought it was kinda neat." According to Faye, "I don't think I would turn it in. I mean I've thought about this a lot. I really don't think that I would choose to be other than I am." And in Mel's experience, "Every now and then I'd start to think about being XY . . . and I think it's kinda neat; it's kinda unique. You know? [It] like sets me apart from everybody else." Despite acknowledging challenges associated with being intersexed, none of the 41 individuals I interviewed expressed that they would rather have been born non-intersexed or not been born at all.

Acknowledging one's difference to oneself and to others is the second part of the coming-out process. Barbara, Martha, and Max speak of the overwhelmingly positive experiences they had at stage two, when they told others about their intersexuality. In Martha's words, "I would recommend [talking about it] to anybody . . . it's a good thing to do. It's the best thing I ever did. I think the more I think about it, the more I read about it, the more I talk about it, the more . . . confirmation it gives me." Max speaks to the importance of having one's experiences and identity validated by externalizing them through coming out: "Nothing has been better for me than telling as many people as possible—telling it to people who mirror it back to me."

Recall that in stage three of the coming-out process individuals seek similar traits and affirmation in others. Faye speaks to the isolation she experienced prior to finding other intersexuals: "Because up until that point I was sure . . . I thought I was the only one." And about the importance of the physical meeting of similar others, Dana said, "Until then I was really alone. I could read all about [intersex]. I could read all the letters and all the papers and all that stuff. But until I met an inter-sexual, they'd still be fictitious, they'd still be this fantasy, this won-drous fantasy. These people that were just like me and who could relate to me and would have compassion for me. For exactly what is causing my pain. [It] was really just a watershed event."

Melody, Claire, and Martha speak to the power of finding out they weren't the only intersexuals after a lifetime of being sure that they would not ever encounter another human being with a body like theirs. In Melody's words, "You can't imagine what it was like! What a relief to find people and not to be alone! It was just incredible. . . . It's like being green in a world of blue and suddenly you find another green person. It was unbelievable. It was just really unbelievable." In Claire's account, "It's been incredibly freeing because there is that sense of . . . not only finding someone like you, but finding a whole community where you belong. . . . There's that wonderful sense of, 'Oh my God; I'm not alone.'" In a very similar conversation, Martha adds, "After having lived all my life in isolation with this, suddenly to hear another person speak the words that I have spoken in the past; share the thoughts that I've had. . . . Well what it felt like was that I've been living on this . . . alien planet, portraying myself, passing myself off as an earthling and I've met someone from, one of my people, from this other planet. You know?"

Joseph exemplifies the fourth stage of coming out: developing pride about one's marginal identity. In his own words, "I mean, think of it . . . what if this was a culture that really honored intersexuals? . . . Really special, really desirable and that then they would be looking, you know, they'd say, 'Don't you think this kid is a hermaphrodite? Oh no, he's a regular one.'"

The "final," fifth stage proposed by many coming-out models is that of integrating one's marginal identity into daily existence. About being able to do just that, Barbara said, "I really have a place in the world. I really am a human being, a very valid human being. It's just wonderful. I am very proud to come out as an AIS person. The world has tried to make us feel like freaks. We have felt like freaks. I felt like a freak most of my life, but look at me. I'm just a human being just like everybody else." Of course, as with any model, linearity is troubling as it signifies a beginning and an end to a far more complex process.

CONCLUSIONS

Based upon this research, it is my conclusion that contemporary attempts to destigmatize intersexuality via surgical and hormonal "sexing" and lack of disclosure do not serve intersexuals or their family members in the manner in which these procedures are intended. I believe that these "sexing" procedures are motivated by a sincere desire to assist intersexuals and their families in achieving social acceptance. The data from my research, however, indicate that the very means intended to normalize are experienced as degrading and shaming.

Given that we lack much extensive follow up on adults who experienced such interventions, certainly more research is needed. My interviews with 41 North American adults serve as an initial database to inform practitioners about their patients' long-term outcome, satisfaction, and quality of life. These findings suggest the need for continued follow up as well as an open dialogue between practitioners and adult intersexuals and their family members regarding how to create a rational and ethical treatment model that will truly exist for the sake of the children.

ACKNOWLEDGMENTS

The author wishes to thank the University of Minnesota's Department of Sociology for the Anna Welsch Bright Memorial Award and the University of Minnesota's Graduate School for a Doctoral Dissertation Fellowship and a Doctoral Dissertation Special Grant.

She also gratefully acknowledges Jeylan T. Mortimer and Walter O. Bockting for their support and guidance, Alice Dreger and Cheryl Chase for their editorial advice, and Christine C. Mack and Lisa K. Mallon for their assistance in transcribing the interviews.

The material presented in this chapter is from "Sexing the Intersexed: Lived Experiences in the Socio-Cultural Context," a research project conducted by Sharon E. Preves, reviewed by the University of Minnesota Research Subjects' Protection Program, Human Subjects Code # 9612S12135, renewed 18 November 1998, Assurance of Compliance # M1337.

NOTES

1. Note: most participants chose to use pseudonyms.

2. R. Hubbard, *The Politics of Women's Biology* (New Brunswick, N.J.: Rutgers University Press, 1990); J. Lorber, *Paradoxes of Gender* (New Haven, Conn.: Yale University Press, 1994).

3. L. Fiedler, *Freaks: Myths and Images of the Secret Self* (New York: Anchor Books, Doubleday, 1978).

4. While the majority of intersex conditions are found to be physiologically benign, some conditions do require surgical or hormonal intervention for the physical health of the individual. Most notably this occurs in cases where elimination of urine and feces is rendered difficult due to the intersexed nature of the body or, in rare cases of salt-wasting congenital adrenal hyperplasia, where hormone therapy is required. See, for example, S. Kessler, *Lessons from the Intersexed* (New Brunswick, N.J.: Rutgers University Press, 1998); and M. Diamond and K. Sigmundson, "Management of Intersexuality: Guidelines for Dealing with Persons with Ambiguous Genitalia," *Archives of Pediatric Adolescent Medicine* 151 (October 1997): 1046-50.

5. J. Butler, *Gender Trouble: Feminism and the Subversion of Identity* (New York: Routledge, 1990); J. Butler, *Bodies that Matter: on the Discursive Limits of "Sex"* (New York: Routledge, 1993); S.J. Kessler and W. McKenna, *Gender: An Ethnomethodological Approach* (University of Chicago Press, 1978); S.L. Bem, *The Lenses of Gender: Transforming the Debate on Sexual Inequality* (New Haven, Conn.: Yale University Press, 1993).

6. Fiedler, *Freaks: Myths and Images of the Secret Self,* see note 3 above.

7. H. Garfinkel, *Studies in Ethnomethodology* (Englewood Cliffs, N.J.: Prentice Hall, 1967).

8. E. Goffman, *Stigma: Notes on the Management of Spoiled Identity* (Englewood Cliffs, N.J.: Prentice-Hall, 1963).

9. J. Money, J.G. Hampson, and J.L. Hampson, "Hermaphroditism: Recommendations Concerning Assignment of Sex, Change of Sex, and Psychologic Management," *Bulletin of the Johns Hopkins Hospital* 97 (1955): 284-300.

10. J. Money, *Sex Errors of the Body: Dilemmas, Education, Counseling* (Baltimore, Md.: Johns Hopkins Press, 1968); J. Money, *Biographies of Gender and Hermaphroditism in Paired Comparisons* (Amsterdam, the Netherlands: Elsevier Science Publishers, 1991); J. Money, *Sex Errors of the Body and Related Syndromes* (Baltimore, Md.: Paul H. Brookes, 1994); J. Money and A. Ehrhardt, *Man & Woman Boy & Girl: Differentiation and Dimorphism of Gender Identity* (Baltimore, Md.: Johns Hopkins University Press, 1972).

11. H. Meyer-Bahlburg, "Gender Assignment in Intersexuality," *Journal of Psychology & Human Sexuality* 10 (1998): 1-21.

12. See, for example, A.D. Dreger, " 'Ambiguous Sex'—or Ambivalent Medicine? Ethical Issues in the Treatment of Intersexuality," *Hastings Center Report* 28, no. 3 (1998): 24-36; C. Elliott, "Why Can't We Go on as Three?" *Hastings*

Center Report 28, no. 3 (1998): 36-39; Kessler, *Lessons from the Intersexed*, see note 4 above; A. Natarajan, "Medical Ethics and Truth Telling in the Case of Androgen Insensitivity," *Canadian Medical Association Journal* 154, no. 4 (1996): 568-70; and B.D. Kemp et al., "Sex, Lies and Androgen Insensitivity Syndrome," *Canadian Medical Association Journal* 154, no. 12 (1996): 1829-33.

13. I have been compiling a list of intersex support network resources throughout North America. Contact information for the 16 groups that I have located follows. They are listed alphabetically:

- **Ambiguous Genitalia Support Network,** P.O. Box 313, Clements, Calif. 95227; telephone: (209) 727-0313
- **Androgen Insensitivity Syndrome (AIS) Support Group Canada,** P.O. Box 425, Postal Station C, 1117 Queen St. West, Toronto, P.Q., M6J 3P5, Canada
- **Androgen Insensitivity Syndrome (AIS) Support Group U.S.,** 4203 Genessee #103-436, San Diego, Calif. 92117-4950; e-mail: < aissg@aol.com >; website: < http://www.medhelp.org/www.ais >
- **Coalition for Intersex Support, Activism, and Education;** P.O. Box 1594, Baltimore, MD 21202; telephone: (410) 235-5146; website: < http://www.sonic.net/ ~ cisae >
- **Congenital Adrenal Hyperplasia Network,** c/o 4182 Mississippi St., San Diego, Calif. 92104
- **Congenital Adrenal Hyperplasia Support Association,** 1302 County Rd. 4, Wrenshall, Minn. 55797; work telephone: (218) 384-3863
- **Hermaphrodite Education and Listening Post (HELP),** P.O. Box 26292, Jacksonville, Fla. 32226; e-mail: < help@southeast.net >; website: < http://www.help@jaxnet.com >
- **Intersex Society of Canada (ISCA),** Box 1076, Haliburton, Ont., K0M 1S0, Canada
- **Intersex Society of North America (ISNA),** P.O. Box 31791, San Francisco, Calif. 94131; e-mail: < info@isna.org >; website: < http://www.isna.org >
- **Intersex Support Group International;** website: < http://www.isgi.org >; e-mail: < care@isgi.org >
- **K.S. & Associates (Klinefelter's Syndrome),** P.O. Box 119, Roseville, Calif. 95661-0119; e-mail: < raylstoc@ix.netcom.com >; website: < http://www.medhelp.org/web/ks.htm >
- The **MAGIC Foundation (Congenital Adrenal Hyperplasia),** 1327 N. Harlem Ave., Oak Park, Ill. 60302; telephone: (708) 383-0808; FAX: (708) 383-0899; Parent Help Line: 800-3 MAGIC 3
- The **Middlesex Group,** P.O. Box 25, Newtonville, Mass. 02460; telephone: (617) 630-9263; e-mail: < themiddlesex@juno.com >
- **National Adrenal Diseases Foundation,** 505 Northern Blvd., Great Neck, N.Y. 11021; website: < http://medhlp.netusa.net/www/nadf.htm >
- **Support and Educational Exchange for Klinefelter's Syndrome (SEEKS),** 1417 25th Avenue Dr. West, Bradenton, Fla. 34205-6449; telephone: (941) 750-8044

• **Turner's Syndrome Society of the U.S.**, 1313 S.E. 5th St., Ste. 327, Minneapolis, Minn. 55414

14. See, for example, A.D. Dreger, *Hermaphrodites and the Medical Invention of Sex* (Cambridge, Mass.: Harvard University Press, 1998); Kessler, *Lessons from the Intersexed,* see note 4 above; Diamond and Sigmundson, "Management of Intersexuality," see note 4 above; and C. Chase, "Hermaphrodites with Attitude: Mapping the Emergence of Intersex Political Activism," *GLQ: A Journal of Lesbian and Gay Studies* 4, no. 2 (1998): 189-211.

15. Of the 41 interviews, 38 were conducted face-to-face; 3 were conducted via telephone.

16. ATLAS/ti, Version 4.1, 1998. Scientific Software Development, Berlin.

17. K. Lebacqz, "Difference or Defect? Intersexuality and the Politics of Difference," *Annual of the Society of Christian Ethics* (1997) 213-29.

18. Natarajan, "Medical Ethics and Truth Telling," see note 12 above.

19. R.R. Anspach, "From Stigma to Identity Politics: Political Activism Among the Physically Disabled and Former Mental Patients," *Social Science & Medicine* 13A (1979): 765-73; D. Barnard, "Healing the Damaged Self: Identity, Intimacy, and Meaning in the Lives of the Chronically Ill," *Perspectives in Biology and Medicine* 33, no. 4 (1990): 535-46; H. Hahn, "Can Disability be Beautiful?" *Social Policy* 18, no. 3 (1988): 26-32; J. Sudsman, "Disability, Stigma and Deviance," *Social Science & Medicine* 38, no. 1 (1994): 15-22; and K.K. Yoshida, "Reshaping the Self: A Pendular Reconstruction of Self and Identity Among Adults with Traumatic Spinal Cord Injury," *Sociology of Health and Illness* 15, no. 2 (1993): 217-45.

20. G. Becker, "Coping with Stigma: Lifelong Adaptation of Deaf People," *Social Science & Medicine* 15B (1981): 21-24.

21. V.C. Cass, "Homosexual Identity Formation: A Theoretical Model," *Journal of Homosexuality* 4 (1979): 219-35; E. Coleman, "Assessment of Sexual Orientation," *Journal of Homosexuality* 14, no. 1/2 (1987): 9-24; and H.L. Minton and G.J. McDonald, "Homosexual Identity Formation as a Developmental Process," *Journal of Homosexuality* 9 (1984): 91-104.

22. S. Stone, "The *Empire* Strikes Back," in *Body Guards: The Cultural Politics of Gender Ambiguity,* ed. J. Epstein and K. Straub (Cambridge, Mass.: Harvard University Press, 1991), 280-304.

23. W.O. Bockting, "Transgender Coming-Out: Implications for the Clinical Management of Gender Dysphoria," *Journal of Gender Studies* 17, no. 1 (1995): 17-20; and W.O. Bockting, "Transgender Coming-Out: Implications for the Clinical Management of Gender Dysphoria," in *Gender Blending,* ed. B. Bullough, V. Bullough, and J. Elias (Amherst, N.Y.: Prometheus Books, 1997).

24. Chase, "Hermaphrodites with Attitude," see note 14 above.

PART 2

Living, Learning, and Loving with Intersex

Introduction to Part 2

While the three other parts of this book also contain first-person narratives of people living with intersex, this sections hones in on the day-to-day lives of intersexed people and their families. The reader is encouraged to notice what about intersex—and especially the medical treatment of it—makes these narratives extraordinary, but also to notice that intersex does not constitute the whole of any intersexed person's life. As these writings show, people who are intersexed have the same basic kinds of desires, needs, concerns, fears, and hopes as everyone else. The photographs included in this section help to achieve the task of these essays—to put a human face on intersex.

Several of the following pieces document the experiences of intersexed people who were not subjected to extensive "normalizing" medical treatments. All the pieces show that, regardless of the intent and methodology of medical procedures, intersex does not disappear when the patient and his/her family leave the clinic.

Many of these essays also remind that intersex is, and always will be, about sex, that is, sexual relations (a fact that can make dealing with intersex in children especially awkward and uncomfortable for some). In their essays, Martha Coventry and Tamara Alexander detail how intersexuality has been a part of their erotic encounters; the remainder of the essays touch more briefly on this topic.

In the end, the autobiographies in this book reveal the central truism that will always make the treatment of intersex challenging: each person experiences it differently. None of these essays should be taken as the definitive statement of what it means to be intersexed or what it means to be the parent or lover of an intersexed person. Instead, collectively they open a window into life with intersex, a window that until recently has been closed and curtained.

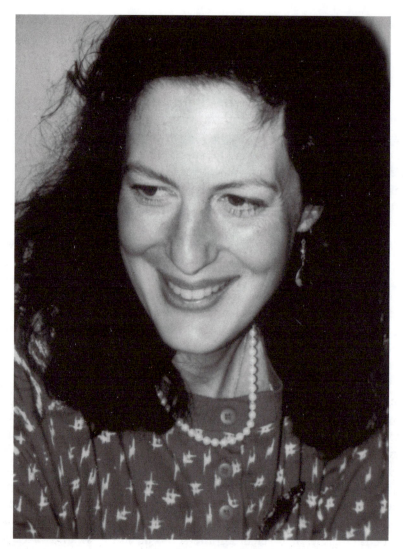

Martha Coventry

5

Finding the Words

Martha Coventry

" . . . your clit with its tongue out waiting for my breath."
—Minnie Bruce Pratt

When I was growing up, and well into adulthood, I used to have a waking nightmare that a squad of men in uniforms would arrive at my door, take me into the night, and execute me for not being a real woman. In my mind, they were always justified and I never raised my voice in protest. In 1987, when my youngest daughter was two and I was 35, I was incapacitated nearly to the point of self-destruction by some unknown shame. I began intensive therapy, desperate to discover why I felt so bad and so wrong. One Sunday morning, feeling inches away from disaster, I called my therapist. "I don't know if this is important," I said shakily, "but I had this operation when I was a child." There. I had said it out loud, and in that instant a tiny sliver of light pierced the dark mystery of my life.

At that point, I knew little of what had been done to me when I was six years old. One November evening in 1958, my mother had come into the bathroom where I was playing in the tub. I had been to the doctor a few days before and men had looked between my legs. She told me that I had to go to the hospital the next day for an operation. I remember something rushing out of me then, like wind through a closing door—all my power escaping. No explanation was given for the surgery, and when the surgeon cut out most of my half-inch clitoris, it was as if he cut out my tongue. I could not cry out to save myself, and that stifled scream wedged in my throat, blocking my voice. Endless fears about who and what I was took the place of words and they settled like a shroud over me.

At age 11 or 12, I had my first orgasm. Somehow I had brought myself to the edge and I just touched the opening to my vagina and it happened. Perhaps it was this new and powerful experience of pleasure from a place that held so much pain that made me determined to find out the truth about my body. A few nights later I crossed the living room, my bare feet on the cool cork squares carrying me towards my parents, the two people who were my only safety. They sat at the dining room table. Big black and white photos of my sisters and me were laid out under the light. My mother picked mine up and I heard the word boy come out of her mouth. Fear heaved in me. I was a boy. I was supposed to be a boy. It was too late to stop myself. "What was that operation I had?" I blurted, as my gut tightened against the blow of the answer. My loving father, a surgeon, looked at me and, with no idea of what his words would do to the rest of my life, said "Don't be so self-examining." The moment of silence that followed that dismissal lasted for almost 25 years.

In warfare there is a technique called sapping. Saps are trenches that are dug underground, silently, beneath an enemy's fortifications. Eventually the walls collapse under their own weight. To be lied to as a child about your own body, to have your life as a sexual being so ignored that you are not even given answers to your questions is to have your heart and soul relentlessly undermined. The thing that makes you wild and free is insidiously crippled. To heal that childhood state of wildness, you have to rescue your own life and learn to speak about who you are. The life you had no power to save when you were 18 months, or six years old, or 13, you have to save at 28, or 36, or 55. You have endless chances. And it is never too late.

I was a grown woman when I started to ask questions again about my body. I was careful this time, protective of this little girl terrified of her own reflection. I had never been sure of my sexual identity and was still afraid that what the surgeon cut off was a penis. I spoke with my father again, asked for my medical records, and listened to my gynecologist read me the summary the hospital sent. My father and my doctor had the same sensible response when I asked what sex I really was: "You had children, isn't that proof enough?" No, as a matter of fact it wasn't. During this time, I went to a resort in Arizona with my husband. I was fragile, with fear and love of myself battling in my head. For a banquet the first night, I wore a low-cut, elegant dress, but my image in the mirror mocked me. My then-short hair did not soften my throat, which seemed masculine and muscular. My arms stuck out hard, sinewy, and tan from my sleeves. I didn't look or feel like a woman. I was in drag. I was a fraud. A mother with two young daughters at home, I spent the entire four days trying to find my way out of believing I was a man. It was as close as I'd come to losing my identity completely and it frightened me back into total and terrified silence. No more questions, no more exploration. I slammed shut and bolted the door that had so briefly and tentatively opened.

Eight years later, I got another chance. I had been fascinated by sex all my life. I started young, playing naked with a girl friend in a sleeping bag, talking another into licking my crotch, being peed on in the woods by a neighbor boy and liking how wrong it felt. My cunt was alive, my scar extra sensitive then to any touch. But wreaking havoc with my budding sexual self was the constant reminder that I was a freak. I was not right in the place where everyone else was perfect. I wanted to be normal. I wanted to fuck. I wanted to be the hippie girl who smoked pot and got screwed everywhere and all the time. The first part came easily, the second part terrified me. The secret I carried about my body stopped every hand as it began its inevitable descent, and cut short every half-naked romp in narrow cabin beds. In high school, it was the sluts I envied, the girls I thought were so free with their bodies. Everything womanly and sexual, even yeast infections, had its allure.

I fell in love my freshman year in college with a kind and safe boy. One night, in bed, I told him about my operation—that I was different from other girls. He looked up from between my legs, said "Oh," and went back to lapping happily away. Our first attempt at intercourse was right out of Sylvia Plath—it hurt, I hated it, and it didn't work. Years later, I married this man and we spent hours together loving each other's bodies, learning to come at the same time using our hands and our mouths. But in this society, and in my mind, it was the old in-and-out that counted. It was my measure of a woman and I was lousy at it. My vagina balked at intercourse, the muscles contracting hard and making it almost impenetrable. Years of fantasizing about sex ended with a new shame. A subtle and ever-so-devastating variation of the old shame: Not only did my body not look like other women's, I couldn't perform like other women.

When the inevitable end came to my marriage, I crashed. It was the response of a woman who was sick to death of being weird, of pretending, of feeling exhausted by a life of envy. Staring me in the face was the unavoidable fact that I was a sexual failure, had never satisfied the man who loved me, and had begun to hate the effort. I narrowly avoided the hospital through the constant attention of my father, my friends, and my therapist, and when I surfaced, I found a raw and beautiful new life waiting for me. The Sufi poet Rumi said that the only way out of the pain is into the pain. I began to stop running from the fear and pain of my life and I turned to embrace them. In the light of a growing affection for myself and my body, they started to lose their power to harm me. Alone much of the time, I would read poetry aloud and sing out in a new strong voice when I walked my dog at night. I started swimming in the nude more and more. I lay in the woods naked, on the earth, in the leaves. I began to crave the feel of my own flawed body, its smells, the taste of its juices. I found new ways of getting pleasure, new ways to come. Sex with myself got noisy and I loved crying out and hearing the sound explode out of me.

In the midst of this love affair with myself, my father died. He was my hero and my most beloved companion. The profound devotion we had for each other is one of the great blessings of my life. To have me clitoridectomized in order to protect me from being "mistaken for a hermaphrodite," as he told me before he died, was not meant as a betrayal of me, but simply one of those most difficult decisions parents make that end up to be wrong. Withholding the truth, when I asked him about myself, was a cruelty he could not understand at the time. Our life together was graced with too much love for bitterness to ever have a chance, but in the end, his death did a surprising thing for me—it cut me loose to finally live my own life and search for my own truths.

Lesbianism had always danced around me. Growing up, I thought that if I were attracted to girls, it would mean I was really a boy. When I read of women who loved women, like Gertrude Stein and Virginia Woolf, I ached at their bravery to claim who they really were. And although I felt an odd bond and natural connection with them, I didn't even dare to play with the possibility of lesbianism myself. And besides, even if the love those women made was strange, their bodies were normal. I put myself again outside the fold. When I was 22, I went into a gay bar with a friend in Quebec City, where I was studying. I was entranced. For the first time, in that dark and smoky place, I saw women dancing pressed up against each other. I went back to my dorm room and cried for the next four months, filled with anguish at my desire to return there and my fear at what it would prove about me. In the 20 years that followed, a sadness lived in me always that I would never know that kind of love. With the end of my marriage, the death of my father, and a growing determination to look squarely at my own life, I had no reasons to hold my desire at bay any longer. I was finally ready to let myself slowly fall into the patiently waiting arms of lesbianism. I will never know the connection between my intersexuality and my homosexuality, but all the queerness I felt growing up finally has a home.

Embracing my love for women not only makes me happy, it is the thing that I had been waiting for to give me the courage to look at my body, and at who and what I truly was, without turning away. I could never have found my intersexual self until I had found and loved my sexual self. A friend introduced me to a new gynecologist—a wise, irreverent man—and he and I explored my body in detail. We prodded and spread, measured and probed with my complete medical records in hand, to understand what I might have looked like and exactly what the surgery had removed. I brought a hunk of clay to his office and we fashioned a model of the vulva I was born with. I began to write vignettes of growing up, of sex, of gender struggles, of madness.

One of the things about being born with genitals that challenge what is considered normal, is that no one ever tells you that there is anyone like you. You feel completely and totally alone. Even today, young children are never put in touch with others who are going through the same thing. You are purposely isolated, your difference covered up—and it is horrible. One day, I met with my writing teacher at her house. Next to my place at the table was a newsletter: *Hermaphrodites with Attitude* was written across the top. Upon seeing that word, which still had the power to terrify me, written so bold, so proud, I became suddenly unable to speak, even to breathe. Reading the text, I found my story in other people's words. People I did not even know existed. It was as if my whole life had been lived to reach just this one moment. I took the newsletter home, and for days and days would pick it up in disbelief and hold it to my chest like a talisman.

And so it started, the strength that comes from finding those like you. The words that used to frighten me, make my skin crawl, like *gender* and *hermaphrodite*, roll off my tongue easier now. They are beginning to belong to me. I will never find the words of my six-year old self, and that is fitting. Today I have the reasoned and educated voice of a grown woman who knows harm when she sees it and is increasingly growing strong enough to name it and try to stop it. Saying this does not mean I am always brave, because I'm not. Speaking out as an intersexual, as a hermaphrodite, I go forward, but I also still retreat to protect myself. At one moment I may tell a friend my story or talk knowledgeably about it on the phone with a stranger. But then the subject comes up in a room full of people, and I speak in generalities, as if it were something that happens to others. And I feel that silence between my legs, the place that sets me and my past apart from most other women. But I'm kind to myself when I can't quite tell the whole truth, as all intersexuals should be. We have lifetimes of shame to overcome and, for most of us, this has been a secret that we have guarded with our lives and at great expense. Coming out as a hermaphrodite has its own precious timing. You can't peel the chrysalis off a butterfly and expect it to survive any more than we can speak out, or even face our own truth, before we are ready.

If you are intersexed, listen to your heart—slowly you will emerge. It takes commitment and courage, it is frightening, but not nearly as frightening as that monster you created all those years out of your own sweet body. As you tell your story and tell it again, a sort of transformation takes place. You start to speak for all intersex people who have ever lived and are yet to be born. Your intensely personal story drops into the background, and what comes forward is your story, as a kind of transcendent truth. Try to love yourself enough to free your hermaphroditic voice, so we can all claim our lives, and the bodies we deserve to celebrate.

ACKNOWLEDGMENT

This chapter first appeared in *Chrysalis: The Journal of Transgressive Gender Identities* 2, no. 5 (Fall 1997/Winter 1998); © 1998 by Martha Coventry; used with permission.

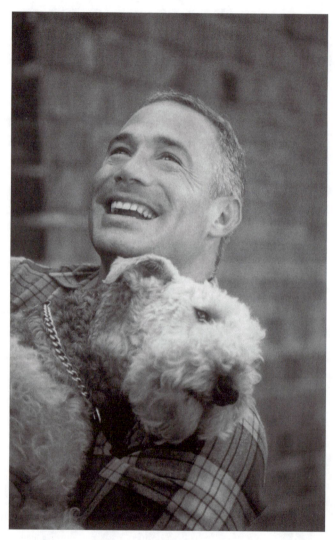

Howard Devore

6

Growing Up in the Surgical Maelstrom

Howard Devore

I'm now 40, and I've done a lot of healing. I am a licensed therapist, and I've used my experience—of being made to suffer unnecessarily by treatment for being intersexual—to make patient advocacy an important aspect of my work. I've healed a great deal through my involvement with the cancer community, where I was able to help people avoid unnecessary medical interventions. And I have studied sex and sexuality, which has been an important element in coming to a place where I can help others, rather than feeling like I was the only one in the world. It also helped me to realize that I could have successful relationships, including sexual relations. A lot of the defeat and depression that I felt growing up left me when I realized that doctors and parents were wrong. They believed that I could not be happy without normal genitals. When I understood that wasn't true, my life completely changed.

It was my mother's job to shuttle me back and forth to the hospital. I've had 16 surgeries on my genitals, and they performed 10 operations by age 10, pretty regularly once a year. It's pretty hard on a father if his son is sexually different, and it's still not easy for my father to discuss.

It was hard on my mother, a typical fifties mom who didn't work. She was the one who had to deal with these teams of high-powered doctors all the time. She's told me what it was like when I was born—the doctor didn't say anything, she looked around and saw the two nurses look down, avoiding eye contact with her. My parents weren't allowed to see me until the doctors had performed lots of tests, and had made up their minds to assign me as male.

My childhood was filled with pain, surgery, skin grafts, and isolation. I remember that when school vacation came, the other kids went somewhere fun. I went to the hospital during vacation, so I wouldn't miss too much school. When vacation was over, I would return to school, often not yet healed from the latest surgery. Sometimes I went back to school with tubes coming out of me, and stitches and scars, and I couldn't walk well. They made arrangements for me to use the teachers' rest room. I have no idea what they told the teachers.

I didn't know any other children who were like me. I asked doctors questions all the time, but they would never tell me anything except to be careful and not to complain. They never told me that there were any other children like me. Other children went on vacation; I went to the hospital. Children, of course, are quick to pick up on difference, and they were very cruel to me. I felt like a freak, an embarrassment, and a burden to my family. But I got the message that I had to pretend everything was OK. The privacy of my hell was something that I had to deal with on my own, and I was very withdrawn and depressed. By the time I was a teenager, I was just hopeless, suicidal. I thought that was a good way out. I let out a little bit of what was going on with me to a friend's mother who was a psychotherapist. She got me in to see someone who evaluated me and saw that I was seriously suicidal.

Early on I had gotten very, very strong warnings not to let other children see me with my clothes off, and particularly not to let them see my genitals. Of course, it was pretty easy for the other kids to pick up on the fact that for years I didn't use the kids' bathroom, or that I couldn't walk well when we came back from vacations. I was lucky that I didn't have to expose my genitals to the other children in elementary school. By junior high, the psychiatrist helped make it possible for me to participate in mandatory gym classes, but not have to shower with other boys. They would have had a great deal of trouble making sense of or understanding what they would have seen. The doctors insist that you can't let a child go to school with ambiguous genitals, but the genitals they created were certainly strange-looking.

Each year they performed surgery on me, and I watched and felt how rapidly the surgery would break down each time. They couldn't have missed it, either—there's no reason for some of the work that they did on me outside of arrogance or incompetence. I spent many years in surgery whose purpose was to make me pee at the end of my penis. If they had just left my urinary meatus [pee-hole] where it was, at the base of my penis right by the scrotum, I could have avoided at least 12 of those surgeries. And it's not just my genitals. They would take large pieces of tissue from other parts of my body to try to create a tube of skin for me to pee through, and those areas are scarred as well.

The tube that most men pee through is not made of skin, it's made of a special kind of tissue that can handle contact with urine, and being continuously moist and warm, without breaking down or becoming infected. The tubes that they made for me out of skin from other parts of my body broke down over and over, and I regularly get bladder infections. And I still have to sit to pee. I have never been without fistulae [holes in the penis where the surgery has broken down], and I've had the entire tube replaced twice, with large skin grafts. If they had just let me pee sitting down, neither I nor my family would have had to suffer all of that—the expense, the pain, the repeated surgeries, the drugs, the repeated tissue breakdowns and urine leaks. It would have been just fine to have a penis that peed out of the bottom instead of the top, and didn't have the feeling damaged.

The promise that you will be able to pee standing up is just plain false, especially when the urinary meatus is at the bottom of the penis. Such a large skin graft can't heal with the blood supply that is available in the genitals. I believe that they know that, but it seems that genital appearance and the promise of normalcy are more important to young parents than a clear-headed acceptance of reality.

ACKNOWLEDGMENT

This chapter first appeared in *Chrysalis: The Journal of Transgressive Gender Identities* 2, no. 5 (Fall 1997/Winter 1998); © 1998 by Howard Devore; used with permission.

7

A Mother's Care

An Interview with "Sue" and "Margaret" by Alice Domurat Dreger and Cheryl Chase

The following are excerpts from an interview conducted by Alice Domurat Dreger and Cheryl Chase with an adult woman, identified here as "Sue," and her mother, identified here as "Margaret." Sue was born with a large clitoris, and against at least one physician's recommendation, Margaret decided not to have a surgeon reduce the size of Sue's clitoris. Margaret came to this decision by following her practice of "examining the doctors." She decided that the doctor who was bothered by Sue's large clitoris was, like Freud, too phallic-centric. Having interviewed her obstetrician, who saw many women with large clitorises, and having been assured by the obstetrician that those women did well, Margaret decided to leave decisions about clitoral surgeries to Sue herself. Sue never chose to reduce her clitoral size, and, in fact, in a recent follow-up discussion, Sue asked Alice to mention that Sue's lovers have found her large clitoris an asset, "a bonus, a wonderful enhancement to our sexual activity."

Margaret: We had a very nice pediatrician—I fell into what my friends had, and didn't have too much experience about interviewing pediatricians. He came to the house, which was unusual. That was in 1959. . . .

Cheryl: And Sue is your second child?

Margaret: The first one was a stillborn. Sue was the first living child . . . Sue was . . . young [when the issue of her clitoris size was raised], but I heard her [in my mind] saying already, "Think twice, Mom, before you do something to me." So that's number one. And, so, one day, the pediatrician said, looking Sue over, "This is a phallus and has to be removed."

Cheryl: So that wasn't when she was born? That was later?

Margaret: That was later. . . . I guess I didn't jump into surgery—and I'm trying to think back . . . my uncles—I had on my father's side, one uncle was a psychiatrist, another one by marriage to my aunt was an ophthalmologist—on my mother's side, my grandfather was an ophthalmologist and one of her brothers was an orthopedic surgeon who was our g.p. for years . . . . My parents couldn't afford [medical care]—and we would go to the clinic with him. And he was avant-garde—in saying, you know, "No antibiotics, not necessary. Don't overdo it. No aspirin." It was kind of, "[Just] go to bed."

So maybe it was that background. My mother had been a nurse—not an R.N.—a volunteer Red Cross nurse in World War I . . . . And, so, she believed more in T.L.C. [tender loving care]—you know, at that time we still got wrapped up in hot things to get the fever out, and that kind of thing—which is coming back in the alternative world. [Laughs.] So, I'm trying to think, you know—how I got to my thinking of not following every doctor. Of course "Dr. Spock" was my bible—Spock children, spoiled brats [laughs]. I think they survived Dr. Spock pretty well! . . . [To her daughter:] You'll have to read Dr. Spock sometime to find out how you were raised.

Anyway, pretty common sense. And my whole tendency has been that way. . . . So when I heard that [that the "phallus had to come off"], I figured, well, let's see, let's evaluate *the doctor*. And it turns out that he was in therapy. Not just psychotherapy, but analysis. So having had an uncle who was trained by Freud, I had a little bit of background on Freud, and figured, well, you know, that's his tendency [to focus on the phallus], and let's not jump into this.

And so I started doing some research as to who knows more about this, and eventually got to Maryland—Johns Hopkins. [She wrote to Hopkins and John Money.] I don't know if I got the letter from him, or from an associate, saying that apparently that's where the research had been done. And the crucial statement to me, that it said, was that "if it's removed there is a risk of losing sensation." So I thought, "Well, let's be *extra* cautious and not jump into this." [Speaking to her daughter:] You read the letter.

Sue: The letter was from an associate who was responding for the original doctor you wrote to, and it just said, "We don't make a decision.

We can't give advice just based on—you know—your statement. We would need to see the patient for our own observation." You know, just a very form letter, not much [information]. I don't even remember the phrase. [Speaking to her mother:] You said you remember it saying that it could cause loss of sensation. . . . I just remember it was so general, and so vague. It didn't specifically recommend surgery, it didn't recommend anything. It just said, "Bring her in for evaluation, we'll be glad to take a look, and decide from there what advice to give you." And you remember a phrase that said. . . .

Margaret: That it can cause loss of sensation. . . . I remember that because it influenced me a lot. . . . So. I decided, well, the person to ask is my obstetrician who sees women at a later stage—who would see [whether] this [a big clitoris] will cause a problem. And, he said he's seen women with all size clitorises and that he hasn't—wasn't aware [of women with big clitorises experiencing problems]. . . .

Now, I don't know, maybe his Catholicism influenced his decision making very much. He was even reluctant when I needed the [birth control] pill for regulatory purposes, and he very reluctantly gave it to me and said it wasn't for birth control. But he said he hadn't [seen problems in women with big clitorises]—as long as she survived the puberty— until she got hair, pubic hair, and that kids wouldn't make fun of her, that would be the main thing, so as long as we didn't make an issue of it, that she was different, then no problem.

She could always have it done at a later time, if, through *her* choice— and, so my decision was not to do anything. So. But, you know, the wise thing was to go to somebody [like a gynecologist] who sees women at a later age—

Alice: Mmm, that was smart!

Margaret: And I don't know whether any obstetrician would say the same thing, but that was his answer. . . . And I guess the approach, in today's world, is even more so, with managed care—I work in a health library . . . and that's being encouraged, to do your own research, because you don't have the time with a doctor, so you should get more information, and write down your questions, so you have everything.

Cheryl: One of the things that surgeons who are doing genital surgery say is that, it would be too traumatizing for the parents, and the parents wouldn't accept the baby, so in order to make certain that the parents will accept and love their child, we have to perform the surgery as early as possible.

Margaret: But they still have to ask the parents, is that right? I mean, they couldn't possibly do it without . . .

Alice: Did you ever regret your decision, to let your daughter decide for herself?

Margaret: Did I regret it? No.

Cheryl [to Sue]: Did you?

Sue: No. No way.

Cheryl: Did you ever think that you wanted to go and get the surgery for yourself?

Sue: Nope. Never occurred to me. I mean, until you started saying [to me] that people in my situation often had this surgery. . . I said, "You gotta be kidding! That's outrageous."

Margaret [to her daughter]: When did you find out that you were different? You had sisters.

Sue: Oh, I knew some—seemed, from comparing myself to them, that I was different. But it wasn't a problem. It wasn't—it was never an issue.

Margaret: We had various differences. We have an adopted boy, and all my girls had umbilical hernias—you know "outies"?—and instead of having penis envy, he had an "outie" envy, because his was an "innie." [All laugh.] So, there were other differences. So that's the important thing—you know, how comfortable are we with differences. And I guess that reflects more—I don't know whether that reflects more liberal thinking—about diversity, and openness to difference, I guess, that goes along with our thinking. So I guess it would be harder to persuade a conservative, a very conservative person. . . .

Cheryl: You said that when Sue was born, they weren't certain exactly at first what sex she was?

Margaret: Well, I guess because of the enlarged clitoris.

Cheryl: How long did it take them to decide?

Margaret: Uh, I think the obstetrician just told me once that he did a chromosome test because he wanted to make sure.

Cheryl: So was it—

Margaret: While she was still in the hospital. I mean, in those days, you got to have five days in the hospital.

Cheryl: So was it a matter of a couple of days until they told you what sex she was?

Margaret: He didn't tell me until, I mean—we knew it was a girl but he wanted to make sure. So I guess, that part he didn't tell me until he had made sure.

Cheryl: And was that disturbing?

Margaret: No, no. [Laughs.] No, I don't know—I get disturbed about other things!

Sue: Nuclear war, famine . . .

Cheryl: Well, physicians who specialize in this insist that not to know for sure what sex your newborn child is would be so utterly traumatizing that it's an unthinkable, that we could let anybody suffer that way longer than about 36 hours.

Margaret: That sounds so arcane. I mean, that sounds really—I mean, that sounds like they're still on the pedestal, where we put them, and that we can't think for ourselves, and that they're making all the decisions for us? This is why I say, I wouldn't ever pick a doctor whose philosophy is that way.

Alice: Could it also have something to do with the fact that you had lost several children before Sue and were relieved to have an essentially healthy child?

Margaret: Did what have to do with . . . ?

Alice: The fact that you weren't that worried about this issue, of her being a little different?

Margaret: Oh no. I'm a worrier. [Laughs.] No, if there's something to worry about—if I find something to worry about, I'll worry about it. I don't recall worrying. There's too much else going on. She seemed perfectly healthy. . . . It was a normal delivery, and so, no, I wouldn't say that I was worried.

And also, you know, I breastfed, and that was not encouraged at the time, it was very hard to do, to keep them from giving her a bottle. They didn't want to wake the mother up. It [breastfeeding] was really fighting the system to a great extent. . . .

Alice: And, did you talk with Sue about her anatomy when she was growing up?

Margaret: No.

Alice: Didn't talk much about it?

Margaret: Never. Never talked about it. She didn't bring it up, and—

Sue: At one point, after I guess I was 14 or 15 or 16, you mentioned that there was—you had faced a decision of whether to have surgery on me or not—and before I met Cheryl, I was aware that you had . . . um, I think it was before you told me—it was in such a casual way, you said, "Um, you know, at one point the doctor told me you'd have to have surgery—or recommended surgery" and you said "I don't think so." And it wasn't—I don't remember the exact sequence of events, but, um . . .

you know, it didn't come as a surprise to you to find out that other people in my situation had undergone surgery.

Margaret: Hmm.

Sue [Speaking to Cheryl]: Do you recall our early conversation and how things unfolded?

Cheryl: I think that we talked about it [a few years before]. . . . And what I remember is that you told me that your mother had just thought about it on her own, and . . . that seemed like for some time, not just on the spot, but that she had thought about it for some time and then decided that it didn't seem like a good idea. And that there were more times when she brought you to the pediatrician as you were growing up that the pediatrician told you, "That's a phallus, and it's going to have to come off." Does that sound . . .?

Sue: That doesn't ring a bell. I remember just very short, casual comments that you [her mother] had made, and when you told me that you had taken [a prescription drug], and, um, and it just seemed like such a low-key issue, I said, "Oh, OK, so that's history, that's a decision you made," and I didn't realize that there was so much pressure put on other people in your situation to have the surgery done until I met Cheryl and she told me—

Margaret: I didn't either—

Sue: . . . that this [having a large clitoris that wasn't shortened surgically] was a rare case.

Margaret: Never came up with any friends, or . . . No, because the point was to low-key it. I mean, she didn't—

[Pause.]

Cheryl: When we talk to doctors who are managing intersexed babies, they just really scoff at the idea that surgeries shouldn't be performed. I mean, one of the things that they say is that the child will be confused about their own sex, and that they will be ashamed, and that they won't be able to be intimate with anybody as they grow up.

Sue: Wrong! [Laughs.]

Margaret: Well, doesn't that depend on size? Wrong, what?

Sue: On all those counts!

Cheryl: Could you elaborate? [Sue and Margaret laugh.]

Sue: Could I elaborate? Yeah. One by one? [Margaret and Sue laugh.] A, I'm not ashamed of my physiology, my anatomy, B, it has not been a detriment at all to any aspect of my development—social, psychological, sexual, or otherwise—and I have no regrets, and no misgivings about how I am. I wouldn't rather be any other way, to tell you the truth. You know, even if I could completely dial in what I wanted to be like, or look like, that would be pretty low on the list of things I'd want to change.

Margaret: Much more important things.

Cheryl: Well, I think though what you just asked me is important—is, "Doesn't it depend on size?" And, I imagine it does depend on size.

Margaret: So, it can't be one size fits all?

Cheryl: I don't think there's anything you can say about everybody, but I think probably a clitoris, if someone is going to have a problem with it, the larger one is going to be more of a problem than a smaller one. . . . There are some people who are born with genitals more ambiguous than Sue's.

Margaret: Well, I guess a lot of it is our mental attitude. Sue's, mine . . . and Daddy's. Some things, I really took the lead in researching. But I don't recall him [Sue's father] objecting to anything. So, we were sort of together on that. So I guess that's the important factor with . . . women. We had to make the decision. Unfortunately some of them take the advice that they're given.

And I'm trying to think whether with any of the kids, being told anything . . . [Another child of hers] was light weight—borderline premature—she was five pounds, 13 ounces, and they wanted to put her in an incubator. But because I was breastfeeding, the doctor managed to keep her out. So it was really the doctor who was cooperative, too. Actually, you know, now I think because we moved into the house when we were still painting, I'm wondering whether the fumes from the painting caused me to go into labor early with [the other child]. I just . . . you know, nowadays, environmental factors can influence—that's a possibility. You [Sue] were normal weight.

Sue [Speaking to Cheryl]: Are you finding any other success stories, or, favorable stories from your research?

Cheryl: We know a couple people who didn't have surgery but not because their parents resisted [like your mother did], just because it didn't happen.

Alice: They just sort of slipped through the system. . . .

ACKNOWLEDGMENT

The material presented in this chapter is from "Autobiographies of Intersexuals and Their Associates," a research project conducted by Alice Domurat Dreger, reviewed by the Michigan State University's University Committee on Research Involving Human Subjects, IRB# 97387, category 2-I.

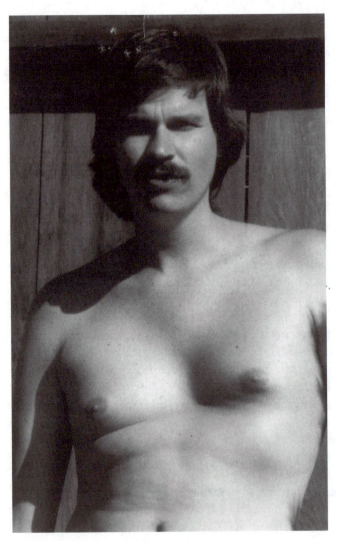

D. Cameron, before testosterone treatment

8

Caught Between:
An Essay on Intersexuality

D. Cameron

It is only fairly recently that I have discovered the term "inter-sexed" and how it relates to my body. I like the term because I prefer more choices than male or female. I think there is a continuum of Male ········ to ········ Female; like shades of gray from black to white. It wasn't until I was 29 years old that a label was put on my physical differences, differences that I never quite understood. I had large nipples on smallish breasts, peanut-size testicles, and cellulite-type hairless fatty tissue over most of my body. I was told at an infertility clinic that I had an extra X chromosome and a karyotype of XXY-47. This is commonly known as Klinefelter's syndrome. I was informed that I was genetically sterile and that my "sex glands" produced only 10 percent of what was considered normal testosterone levels for a male. I was advised to immediately start testosterone replacement therapy. I was told that my "sex drive would increase," I would "gain weight and my shoulders would broaden," and that I would have to do this every two weeks for the rest of my life. The medical journals called my condition "feminized male." I had always felt caught between the sexes without knowing why.

This reality was not evident at my birth in 1947. When puberty came, I knew I was different from other boys. I was often teased for having small testicles, and I had gynecomastia (breast growth in a male). It was an awkward time for me as I was very tall (six feet, nine inches, at 15 years old). As I now have learned, testosterone is needed to stop the

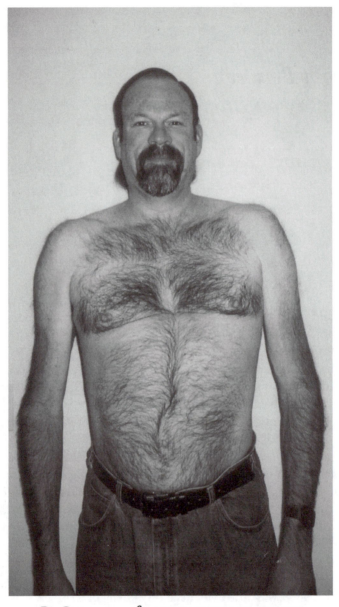

D. Cameron, after testosterone treatment

growth of the long bones, in arms and legs. I was a self-conscious, sensitive, and emotional kid. My mother was concerned about the lack of
development and after several visits the doctor (incorrectly) assured her
that I would grow up "normal" and that I could produce children.

Not having any other information or knowledge about my situation, at the advice of the doctor at the fertility clinic, I faithfully got my
300 mg. injections of testosterone every two weeks. I soon found myself
going through puberty all over again—in my early thirties. I was a first
tenor turning into a baritone. I began shaving, and eventually grew a
beard. Hair sprouted everywhere on my once smooth body. There were
phenomenal changes for me, both physically and psychologically. The
greatest change was having so much sexual energy. For the first time I
appreciated what the word "horny" meant.

During this period (1976-1981), I did not have any counseling for
emotional issues. My main support came from my life-partner, Peter,
whom I met in 1978. I dealt with most of my "transformation" alone.

The first few years of testosterone replacement therapy, I had the
sensation of "reverse menopause" combined with the feeling that my
female persona was dying. It was an overwhelming time of confusion,
yet the confusion was mixed with discovery. I didn't understand why I
had been chosen to have this experience in my life, and wondered whether
I should instead have stayed who I was. In the end, because I was so tall,
I decided to proceed, in order to find out what being "male" was like. I
often regret that decision. When I first moved to San Francisco in 1979,
I got my injections at Kaiser Hospital, but by 1983 I had learned how to
inject myself. I would have to get into a semi-yoga position to push the
large needle intramuscularly into my buttocks.

For the next 10 years I became quite strong and trim. I exchanged
sedentary employment for more physically challenging work, and started
my own home and garden renovation business. By now my once hairless body was covered—much to my dismay—with hair, and my head
was beginning to bald. I did not realize that these were side-effects of
testosterone replacement therapy. Now my body appeared very masculine and I was told that, to further "improve the effect," I could have
testicular implants and have my breast tissue removed. I chose not to
have surgery.

In 1991, my sex drive began to diminish significantly. I feared that
my testosterone replacement therapy had failed. I started to think of the
testosterone as a poison in my system. I started to get back in touch with
my female side—and realized that I had never completely lost her. Emo-

tionally and spiritually, I have always felt more feminine, and I began to doubt the correctness of the decision I had taken, in 1976, to find out what being male was like. My sexual orientation had not changed—I was still attracted to men. I considered lowering my hormone dosage, but doctors advised against it. There would be serious side-effects, they told me. But could the side-effects be anymore painful than the fear of prostate, breast, or testicular cancer by continuing the injections, I wondered? Why wasn't I told any of this when I started hormone therapy? Have I become a "virilized female"? (Not unlike a female-to-male transsexual with a penis?) I felt caught between again.

For two or three years, my doctor raised my testosterone dosage to 350 to 400 mg. every two weeks to see if that would improve my sex drive. My sex drive was unchanged, but I started having more prostate and urinary problems. I was put on another drug to try to compensate for the side-effects of the testosterone.

In October 1995, I attended the first national conference of K.S. & Associates (a Klinefelter's syndrome support group) in Washington, D.C. The conference was a disappointment to me, in that intersex and gender issues were never discussed. I assumed this was probably due to what I perceived as homophobia on the part of the group's founders (who are parents of children with Klinefelter's syndrome) and of the supporting staff of Johns Hopkins Hospital. There was a small group panel that was supposed to discuss gender, but instead they discussed sexual orientation. The panel immediately became polarized and did not move forward. There were about 80 people with Klinefelter's attending, including quite a few children. Some 20 of us adults spotted each other as queer, and got together spontaneously to discuss our sexuality and our disappointment over the lack of support by K.S. & Associates for gender issues.

At that conference, I learned that the U.S. Food and Drug Administration had just approved the Androderm patch, a method of delivering testosterone without injection. I was unable to wear the Testoderm patch because my scrotum is so small that it does not provide enough area for the patch to work. In December 1995, I decided to stop my injections as they had become painful and I needed a rest after 19 years. (When I stopped the injections, I was up to 350 mg. every two weeks.) Some side-effects occurred within five weeks: fatigue, mood swings, depression, more difficulty urinating. I had my testosterone level checked. It was 12 (normal male levels are 400 to 1,100). I realized that I could not return to where I was in 1976, before the testosterone injections, and decided that it was best to stay on the journey I had started. Somehow I would cope. I knew that being "caught between" would be my life challenge, and that would be OK, since I felt whole with all my unique parts. I needed to treasure my "X"ception.

In January of 1996 I returned to testosterone therapy, with one Androderm patch a day. My energy improved, but flattened out in two weeks. Three weeks later I began wearing the recommended two patches to see if my moods and depression would improve. I endured Androderm patches for five months. It was strange adjusting to wearing patches. They must be changed once a day and cannot be worn on the same site again for seven days. You rotate the placement, with preferred sites being upper arm, back, thigh or abdomen. They are about three inches in diameter and have white rings around the circumference of the adhering portion. Wearing them, I felt self-conscious at the gym and in the shower. The last thing I wanted to do was draw more attention to myself.

Because of the patches I had constant skin rashes and itchiness that I had to use hydrocortisone cream to heal. The adhesive from the patch was so gummy that only a pumice stone would remove it. Daily I was reminded that I was different and I tried to adjust to this experience. At times I had several splotches of red circles on my skin. Over time, applying the patches to my back, abdomen, upper arms, and occasionally my thighs caused my skin in these places to become too sensitive. My front thighs became the "preferred" site, although to keep the patches on I would have to shave my hair off. After four months of wearing two patches every 24 hours, I had my testosterone level checked and it was only 345. I had expected a higher level and was not motivated to use a third patch.

The main side-effects from the Androderm patch were the development of two large fat deposits, one on the back of my neck, a "buffalo hump" (my adrenal and thyroid gland tests were normal), and the other in the form of a spare tire under my navel. I'm sure this was due to my ingestion of hormones and changes in my hormone ratios. My moods were somewhat altered and I felt more depressed during this five-month period.

Painful injections started looking good again. At least I only had to deal with them every two weeks and they were virtually "garbage" free. I felt "caught between" yet again. I decided that this had to end, that I needed more control over my own destiny. My sex drive was still absent even with the patch, and so I wondered how unfortunate all this hormone replacement therapy had been, since my lack of sex drive was the main reason I originally started on the hormones.

On Father's Day I decided that I had had enough of the patches. I decided to return to injections and wait to see if the medical community would ever come up with an acceptable alternative. I injected 200 mg. of testosterone enanthate into my glutes. It actually felt good! I have had two shots since then, both at 250 mg., and I will stay at this level indefinitely. My energy level has returned as has my sex drive, and I generally feel very good. I do not miss the hassle of patches at all.

Having gone through the writing of this, I realize that this is an important educational opportunity. There are many courageous intersexed people on our planet, not just males and females. Our sex hormones define us or set us free from categories. When others look at me they probably see a big, hairy, bearded man. But I know the TRUTH. I will strive to continue to redefine myself.

My body feels more androgynous, and I am adjusting to the reality of my fat deposits. I guess we are all a combination of male and female, and muscle and fat. I'm allowing my emotions to flow again and am adjusting to another stage of my intersexed being. I no longer feel "caught between." I am a unique blend of my female and male essences, and I expect to continue evolving on that level.

ACKNOWLEDGMENT

This chapter first appeared in *Chrysalis: The Journal of Transgressive Gender Identities* 2, no. 5 (Fall 1997/Winter 1998); © 1998 by D. Cameron; used with permission.

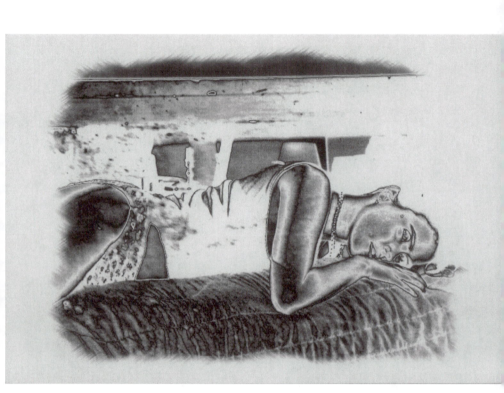

Kim

9

As Is

Kim

I remember laying in bed late one night after my partner and I made love, my clitoris still feeling the warmth and wetness of the inside of her vagina. It felt good. But I wondered, "Am I the only woman who has done this? Am I the only woman whose clitoris knows the feeling of penetration?"

I thought I had discovered the answer while reading a magazine this summer. I read about a woman who was born with a large clitoris like mine. It turned out this woman was Cheryl Chase, and as I read on I found out that hers had been amputated by doctors when she was a child. While this article didn't fulfill my desire to relate with another woman like me, it did introduce me to the word "intersex" and what it might mean to me.

In a further search for understanding, I read through huge medical volumes with black and white photos of infants, like insects tacked to a board for study. And to my dismay, most of these photos were followed by an image of their surgical "correction." The clitoris was removed and only space remained where beauty once grew, like a forest being clear cut and left with only stumps, empty and desolate. I was thinking about how it would feel to touch that unresponsive flesh . . . thinking about how it would feel if that flesh were between my own legs . . . thinking about how another fraction of an inch could have destined me to the same fate.

All this talk about surgery made me wonder what makes doctors so certain that women want a small clitoris, and want it badly enough to sacrifice sexual responsiveness to alter it. In a society where men pride themselves on possessing a large penis, why would women view their bodies so differently? Whose perception of beauty and attractiveness are surgeons basing these decisions on?

Of course I was teased about my body when I was growing up, as is the experience of most children, but that is no reason to alter one's body. A couple of my lovers have teased me tenderly about my androgynous body, and I used to be embarrassed about the way my clitoris stuck out—it didn't hide behind my labia like I thought it should—but again that is no reason to surgically alter it. As an adult I have grown to like my body the way it is. I like the fact that we are each unique individuals, which necessitates a wide variety of body shapes, sizes, and colors. I certainly don't feel the medical establishment has the right to determine which of our bodies are socially acceptable.

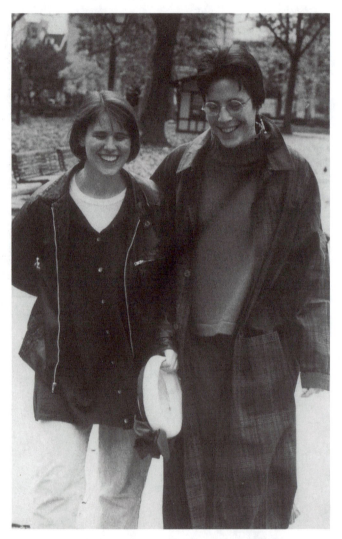

Tamara Alexander and Max Beck

10

Silence = Death

Tamara Alexander

I have been typing and writing the introductory paragraph of this story for several days now, and I keep arriving in the same place. It is hard to get the pieces in place, because creating this picture has been like trying to assemble a thousand-piece jigsaw puzzle in the dark: leave out or misplace one fragment and the picture no longer makes sense. Then there is the difficulty of where to begin. . . .

We met in college, the first day of the spring semester, junior year. Having had an earlier class in that room, I stayed on. She was the first to arrive. Our eyes met across an empty classroom. . . . The neon signboard in my head lit up: something was forever changed. I would spend the next two years chasing down the mystery behind that moment. Love at first sight? Nonsense. Soul mates? Ridiculous. But. . . .

We became friends. Dinners at each other's houses. Study groups. Movie marathons. We even had a date . . . candlelight and wine, out alone, glowing at each other across the table. And I told myself that I had been wrong, that she was straight. . . . Hell, she even got married. I resolved to live with that. It wasn't until April of the following year that I finally told her about the one and only love affair I'd ever had with a woman, and she responded in kind. I thought that this bit of history must have been what I'd been reading when we first met: not that she didn't have feelings for women, just that they had not been about me. How could I have known how wrong I would be?

I returned home to Georgia after graduation. I held her hand in the procession and reminded myself that this was where it ended. She was happily married, and I was . . . adrift. We started a correspondence, ostensibly because she had missed out on having someone to talk to when she was figuring out her sexual orientation and wanted to be that person for me. She was finally talking to me, after two years, about being a lesbian. Need I say that this correspondence took some dangerous turns?

I was mad about her and always had been, and she was telling me her life story. About how she ran away to California in her senior year of college and got embroiled in a lesbian love triangle. About why she married Harold. Oh, and by the way . . . she thought I was beautiful. I wrote back that when I had first met her, I'd been equally enamored. Letters flew on a one-day turnaround. I was sleeping with her letters under my pillow without really understanding why.

We were peeling the onion, one layer at a time.

In my confusion, I reunited with my ex. It was only then that she wrote to tell me how involved she really had been, how deeply it hurt her to have missed our chance, how badly she really had wanted to be with me. I wrote back that I loved her. That I expected to live with the ache of that regret for the rest of my life. I was with Jenny and intended to be, but I could not help but hope our paths would cross again. I sent her Robert Frost's "The Road Not Taken," copying it out by hand on the back of the envelope sitting on the floor of a bookstore. She left Harold.

We fell out of touch. Three months later I spent an entire day thinking of her, and came home to find a book of poetry she had sent. "You can control it," she quoted one of Margaret Atwood's characters, "You can make yourself stop loving someone." The other responded: "That is such horseshit!" The jig was up.

We spoke at all hours of the day over the next two weeks. I called her at work. "I need to come see you." I had expected her excitement, joy, anticipation. She sighed. Her tone was ominous. "Okay," she said. "Come. We'll talk. There are some things you should know about me." "That sounds serious," I said. She agreed: "It is." My first thought was that she had cancer. My next thought was much closer to the mark.

The visit was to be two weeks later. The topic kept coming back up: things that I should know about her. She didn't want to talk about it over the phone. Panic would break into her voice at the subject. "Why are you so afraid to tell me?" I asked. "Nothing could change the way I feel about you." "This could," she said. "It's horrid." Eventually the strain of not talking about it won out, and she told me. By this time, I was already fairly certain what she was going to say.

"When I was born, the doctors couldn't tell whether I was a boy or a girl. . . . " She dictated the speech as if she'd told it many times before and all of the emotion had fallen right out of it. I finally heard the complete story of her college affair with a woman and the six words she said in bed that altered the entire course of Max's life: "Boy, Jude, you sure are weird." Max told me she knew then that she was a lesbian but she could not be with women because they would know how her body was different. She married Harold because men were just less sensitive to the subtleties of women's anatomy.

My response was tears: "I can't believe you've been carrying this around by yourself your whole life." I hadn't been surprised; growing up in a house full of medical texts had acquainted me with intersexuality. I was not, as she had feared, horrified, repulsed, or anxious.

What did you think, she asked me in the car as I was preparing to write this essay about loving her, what did you expect my body to be like? "I thought it would be mysterious and wonderful," I told her. "And it was."

I went up to Philadelphia for four short days over her birthday in February. We attempted to cook, burned the butter, and collapsed in each other's arms on the floor. We left the house only to pick up takeout and Ben & Jerry's Wavy Gravy ice cream. Nonetheless, for the first two nights, she would not take off her boxer shorts. I could feel the wonder of her hardened clit pressing up between my legs through the flannel, but I was not allowed to touch. Although the rest of her body lay out before me to be charted, her cunt was a zealously guarded region. She told me she couldn't lubricate because of the scar tissue, and because the surgeons had taken her labia to make a vaginal opening when she was 15. "Lots of women can't lubricate," I told her. "That's why they make feminine lubricants. There's at least three on the market."

We decided to go shopping. In the feminine hygiene aisle, we compared the relative merits of Gyne-Moistrin and its competitors. I was carefully examining the quality, price, and recommendations of each when I looked up at Max. Her eyes were wide and glazed. She was shaking. Her breath was irregular. I picked up the nearest product, sent her outside to wait, and paid at the register. We went home.

That night we slept downstairs in front of the fire. It was February fifth, her 29th birthday. There was easily a foot of snow on the ground and it had all frozen over. Only her boxers still remained between us.

Later that night she went upstairs to the bathroom, and when she slipped back under the covers, my hands slid from one end of her body to another. The boxers were gone. I will never be able to recapture the magic of that moment. "Ohhh. . . . " She was terrified, and I was aware of her fear and the cost of offering herself up to me in that moment. . . . I have never wanted to pleasure someone, never wanted to offer my hands and my fingers to heal and to love and to delight. . . . I have never been so awed by the feeling of touching as I was that night. I wanted to stroke and explore and learn and know every inch of her, her large and proud clit, the lines and crevasses from scars and healings, the tight cavern of her cunt that held my fingers so tightly. She pulled me down on top of her and wrapped her arms around me and came, calling my name, sobbing against my shoulder. And I wept with her.

I wept for the loss of what she hadn't had and the lovers who hadn't reveled in the wonder of her body, wept for what I hadn't had before I held her in love, and I am weeping as I write this now.

It was a full year before she let me touch her that way again . . . January 17th. Our one-year anniversary. The boxer shorts had been long gone, but most of our lovemaking was by full body contact, tribadism, pressured touch. We made love that anniversary night, and I asked: please. Please let me touch you. Please don't shut me out. Please just lie back and let me love you, the way I want to, the way you deserve to be loved. Let me know you. Let me look. Let me run my tongue into the places you haven't let me before. Let me celebrate you, because I love this, and this, and this. I don't love you despite your differences, I love you because of them. I want you to be this way. I want to enjoy your being this way, because it is good, lovely, delicious. Let me.

And she let me feel her, let me bury my face in her cunt and smell the rich scent of her. Let me slide my tongue over her aching clit and along the entry to her vagina, let me stroke and tease and caress with my fingers. She came in a gush, spilling out over me and the bed. And there were more tears for this ritual, more love, and more letting go. A full year. We were still taking baby steps toward completely open lovemaking. Still peeling onions.

We moved to Atlanta in the summer of 1995. Broken by the stresses of new jobs, financial worries, lack of friends and supports, and a 1912 bungalow which we loved but could barely afford renovating—Max lapsed into a depression. She began to tell me that she was a monster and she just shouldn't be here. The day she did not go to work because she was planning to hang herself, I took her to the hospital. It was the hardest thing I have ever done in my life.

I had the unenviable task of surrendering the illusion that my uncon-
ditional love and acceptance were going to save her. No matter how
much I loved her, no matter what I would give to heal her, I was not
enough. I could not keep her safe. I could not erase 30 years of grief and
doubt about her worth and her place in this world.

I was isolated from other people in ways I hadn't been before; no
one knew her past medical history, and she was not ready for me to talk
to anyone else about it. My friends from Philly called to check on me;
they loved me and understood only that I was in agony because Max was
depressed. They assured me that she would get better, that she would
come home to me and the beautiful life we had created together. I was
not certain she could ever recover from the damage that had been done.

I read her medical records over and over. Sorted through John
Money's articles left from college psych classes. Read her journal, trying
to understand. At night, I screamed my lungs out at the sheer futility of
trying to help her. I had nightmares of surgeons wielding shiny scalpels
tying her down and rearranging her body. I wept at work. I wept at
home. I did endless battle with our mounting financial doom: the mortgage was late, the car unpaid, utilities coming due . . . all without her
income. How would I ever keep things intact so that she had a life to
return to when (IF) she recovered?

Why was there no one to talk to? Why was she sleeping in a tiny bed
in a hospital corridor with hourly safety checks instead of at home with
me? What had I done to merit losing her this way? How could she think
she was bad when I loved her so much? How could she not know how
amazing and special she was?

Life became a parade of visiting hours, drive-thru hamburgers at
Wendy's on the way home, buying her books, taking her Joshua bear,
keeping her family at bay so that she could rest. I was spending all of my
time being busy, painting the room that had been the final stressor, bor-
rowing cash, calling on all of her breaks to check in. For the first weeks,
I only cried. I railed at my therapist about the injustice of life. I mourned
that I couldn't be the one to save her. I could only hold her hand, tell her
to hold on, and pray.

I read her records. . . . And I wondered, if this had happened to me,
if my body had been desecrated and abused and held up in public for the
amusement of interns, would I have survived it even half as well as she
had? Would I have had the courage to go on for 30 years with the memory
of those rapes, my mother's shame and my own, and the lies of doctors?
A lesser person would not still be in the world. I do not think I would
have survived this. No, I know I would not have.

I made promises to keep myself sane. I swore that I would not lose her. I swore that I would not allow this to happen to anyone else. I promised myself that if she slid off the face of this earth out of the exhaustion of fighting for her right to exist, I would not allow this to happen to any child like her. I would find out how and by whom this awful process was being perpetuated, and I would make it stop. I would become louder and louder until I could not be ignored. I have never doubted that I could be a force to be reckoned with, and I was finding out by juggling my whole life those months that I was indeed incredibly strong and capable, and that I could accomplish miracles out of my love for her.

It took four months. Three hospitalizations. Persistent suicidal ideation and unwavering depression. She lost her job because she couldn't stop crying. I dragged her to monthly support group meetings in the gender community. I made her return calls to Cheryl Chase at ISNA. I pushed her to call the people Cheryl sent out to make contact with her. Each time, she would feel a little less alone, and a little more hopeful. And then the depression would creep back, telling her to give up. Telling her she would never be whole, would never be accepted, would never be anything but a shameful secret. As many times as I had learned in that first precious year together that love is an amazing healer, I had still to learn that sometimes shame and blatant evil can be stronger. I might love her with all my heart, but that was one small glow against the bitterness and dark of the rest of her experiences. Would it be enough?

It is now almost a year since that last depression. It still creeps up on us from time to time. When she doesn't come home on time, I have to pace myself not to panic. I have to remind myself that not being home does not mean she has killed herself. But the danger is always there. It's only in the last few weeks that it feels less close, less powerful than me. Less powerful that the sense of self I'm amazed and awed to watch her discover.

She has cut her hair, embraced butch, and found a good endocrinologist. We marched together in the parade at gay pride. I have come to believe myself a part of this community. I may not be transgendered, transsexual, or intersexed. I may have been fortunate enough to be born into a body that matches my sense of self and is accepted by society in its original form. But this is still my fight.

There is a popular slogan in the gay community that proclaims "Silence = Death." Her silence, and mine, almost meant her death. I am reminded of the words of the Catholic priest who recalled that during the holocaust he did not speak because he was not a member of any of the groups they were rounding up for execution. When they came for him, there was no one left to speak for him.

She is my partner, my lover, the greatest gift life ever gave me. I choose to honor her decision to stay alive. I choose to speak on a daily basis. I honor her courage and her complexity. If she walks between the worlds set up by a gender-dichotomous society, then that is where my path leads as well.

A postscript: This piece was written in 1996. Since that time, Max has been living as an out intersexual. He chose to transition to a male gender role in 1998, and is happier than he has ever been.

ACKNOWLEDGMENTS

This chapter first appeared in *Chrysalis: The Journal of Transgressive Gender Identities* 2, no. 5 (Fall 1997/Winter 1998); © 1998 by Tamara Alexander; used with permission. Photo used with the permission of Max Beck.

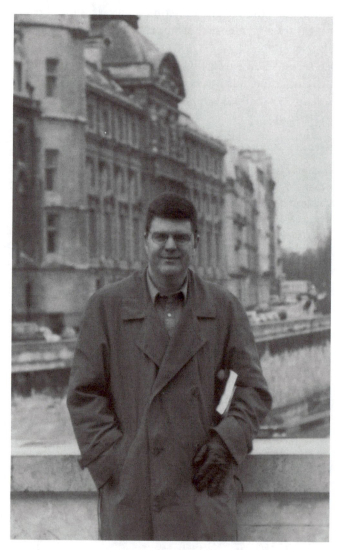

Hale Hawbecker

11

"Who Did This to You?"

Hale Hawbecker

I was born in the early 1960s in Gary, Indiana. My penis was very small (less than an inch long) and my testes were undescended. The doctors told my parents that with such small genitalia it would be impossible for me to function as a male and that surgery had to be performed so that I could be raised as a girl. Fortunately, my parents refused to consent to this. They saw what appeared to be male genitalia and they insisted in knowing my genetic make-up. I was a genetic male, and a perfectly healthy baby. My parents demanded to be allowed to take me home despite the furtive concern of the attending doctors.

When I was two, after a routine physical, the doctors insisted on exploratory surgery to search for my undescended testes. They found them between the kidneys and groin. They removed them, thinking them to be nonfunctional and that they would become cancerous if they remained inside of me. This was a mistake. I have learned as an adult that I have Kallman's syndrome, a condition where the hypothalamus does not stimulate the pituitary to release necessary hormones to stimulate testicular growth. I do not have a sense of smell, a strong indication of Kallman's. Kallman's can be treated by using a device similar to an insulin pump to perform the function of the hypothalamus. The majority of Kallman's syndrome patients are fertile with this treatment. Of course, in my case, this treatment was not possible because the doctors unnecessarily removed my testicles.

Although doctors tried to convince my parents that I would be miserable living as a man with such small genitalia, their fears have not been my life story. True, I have always been very wary undressing in front of others. This was particularly hard in junior high school gym class, and I remember going to class early and running extra laps so that I was the last to use the shower. I sometimes skipped showers altogether if I thought I could get away with it. Even today I am wary showering in a public setting, for instance, in the gym after I work out. But I haven't been naked in front of others enough for this to ever be a huge issue in my life. I just won't join a nudist colony and my genitals will never be much of a factor as to how I interact with other people. And if people reject me for who I am, well, I am better off without them anyway.

As a matter of fact, the only real angst that I have suffered over my genitals has been at the hand of medical professionals. Whenever I went in for examinations as a child and later when I started hormonal treatment, doctors seemed to be perversely fascinated with my genitalia. They would make me sit in frog-legged position, and invite teams of earnest interns to come in and look at me while I was naked on the cold metal examination table, the shame on my face unnoticed by them as they talked about me in the third person and looked at me close, peering at me as if I were a bug under a microscope. Once, I remember I went in for a physical for a scouting camping trip, and the doctor stared in horror at my genitalia and blurted out, "Who did this to you?"—words that still ring in my ears and make me feel mortified 25 years later.

But frankly, as an adult, I do not spend a lot of time concerned about my genitalia. My penis, although small especially when it is not erect, does every thing that I want it to do. It allows me to urinate standing up. It brings me and my partner a great deal of pleasure. It grows erect, it penetrates her vagina, it ejaculates. I don't know what else I need it to do. I am just so lucky that I was able to keep it. Many in my condition were not deemed adequate, and doctors didn't let them keep their genitalia intact. I am shocked that now, over 35 years later, U.S. doctors are still surgically cutting away genitals that don't meet their strict criteria. It seems like something out of Nazi Germany to me. I have pledged to fight this with all I have for the rest of my life.

I am a very good life partner. I am faithful, long-term. I write poetry and am very funny. I have learned to compensate with a lot of creative play and non-penetrative techniques, pleasuring my lover orally, with massage, with sex play, and just spending a lot of time letting her know how thankful I am for every moment I have with her.

And my small genitalia have not really negatively impacted me in any other way that I can think of. I am a successful attorney with a good salary. I identify as a man, and do not have a difficult time playing the part. As a matter of fact, I am actually glad that I was born the way that I was. I view it as a secret challenge that I have overcome, like climbing Everest; it has given me a lot of self-esteem, to know that I have not let my physical condition negatively affect me, and that I have not used it to claim any special victim status either. I get a kick out of it when a male friend says, "Hale, you have balls." I have been tempted to laugh and tell him, "No I don't, actually, but then I have not really missed them much either." There are a lot of things that could have happened to me that would have been a lot worse. My physical condition has not stopped me from enjoying the truly wonderful things in life—a perfect sunset, a sumptuous meal, the laughter of a close friend, or the softness of my lover's kiss. I am glad to be who I am.

PART 3

Changing Perspectives
of the Clinic

Introduction to Part 3

This section includes the two basic clinical perspectives: those of physicians treating intersex; and those of patients who have been treated by intersex specialists.

In the first essay, Bruce Wilson and William Reiner (both specialist physicians who work with intersexed children and their families) trace the shift from the older and now widely criticized paradigm of intersex management to the emerging new paradigm. Their proposed new paradigm attempts to address the ethical and pragmatic problems of the older system, problems highlighted especially in parts 1 and 2 of this book.

In keeping with the focus on the clinic, part 3 continues with two autobiographical essays, by Angela Moreno and Kiira Triea. Both of these life stories bring into full view the need for the paradigm revision for which Wilson and Reiner call. Lest readers assume that the dissatisfied intersexual ex-patients writing in this volume reflect decades gone by, when surgery had yet to be perfected, we should note that Moreno's clitorectomy happened in 1985 at a major urban medical center.

Indeed, Cheryl Chase, a long-time critic of intersex medical management, addresses the common response "surgery is better now" in her aptly titled essay, "Surgical Progress Is Not the Answer to Intersexuality." After showing that current-day surgery has not in fact been demonstrated to be substantially better than past surgeries, Chase argues that the ethical principles of autonomy and informed consent cannot be violated, no matter how much better surgery may become.

Finally, Justine Marut Schober, a surgeon who treats intersexed children, responds to five of the most common criticisms leveled against the published standards for treatment.

12

Management of Intersex:
A Shifting Paradigm

Bruce E. Wilson and William G. Reiner

Picture this scenario: A pediatric endocrinologist refers an eight-year-old "intersexed" girl with XY gonadal dysgenesis (a condition with female external appearance despite "male" chromosomes; see below) to a pediatric surgeon for evaluation of her urinary incontinence. The surgeon's examination and cystoscopy show an urethrocele and an urethrovaginal fistula (anatomic abnormalities of the urethra and vagina). If these abnormalities were not corrected, the girl might suffer recurrent, potentially debilitating urinary tract infections. So, the surgeon schedules and performs an operation to correct the medically problematic urinary tract abnormalities that had concerned the endocrinologist. But, at the same time, the surgeon also performs a colovaginoplasty and a clitoroplasty—in other words, he builds the girl a "vagina" out of part of her colon and he performs cosmetic surgery to reduce and reposition her clitoris. Upon receiving the operative report and learning of the colovaginoplasty and the clitoroplasty, the pediatric endocrinologist becomes very upset. Why?

The above scenario actually happened; one of the authors (BEW) was the referring endocrinologist. This case illustrates the evolving shift now taking place in the paradigm by which children with intersex are managed, and the surgeon mentioned above and the authors stand on opposite sides of the management chasm created by this paradigm shift. Before we discuss the shift and the issues behind it, let us introduce some key background terminology and concepts.

TYPES OF SEX

To understand the conditions that have come to be termed "intersex," one must first realize that sex and gender are not as simple as we think when we typically use the terms "male" and "female." We have tabulated some of the types of sex and gender determination that one can make; note that they can cascade from one to another and that there can be, in some individuals—including intersexuals and transsexuals—contradictions between levels (see table 12-1).

The phrase *genetic sex* usually refers to the presence or absence of the genetic sequence for testicular development. This appears to be the SRY gene on the short arm of the Y chromosome. *Chromosomal sex,* by contrast, is usually defined by the presence or absence of the Y chromosome; most people think of the Y chromosome as the male sex chromosome, so people without a Y chromosome are usually thought of as "genetically female." However, cases of individuals with XX chromosomes, testes, and normal male phenotypes have been reported. In these individuals, the SRY gene has been translocated onto an X or other chromosome. Thus there can be a distinction between genetic sex and chromosomal sex.

Gonadal sex is used to describe the status of the gonads themselves: testicular tissue (either in the form of testes or streaks) indicates a male sex; ovarian tissue indicates a female. Since the late 19th century, medical experts have termed individuals with both ovarian and testicular elements

---

Table 12-1
Some Types of Sex and Gender Determination that Can Be Made

Types

Genetic sex
Chromosomal sex
Gonadal sex
Phenotypic sex (internal)
Phenotypic sex (external)
Sex of rearing
Gender (childhood)
Gender (adulthood)

true hermaphrodites, individuals with ovarian tissue only and "ambiguous" genitalia *female pseudohermaphrodites*, and individuals with testicular tissue only and "ambiguous" genitalia *male pseudohermaphrodites*.[1]

During and after embryonic life, the hormones secreted by the gonadal tissue contribute to the phenotypic (gross anatomical) sex. Muellerian inhibiting factor (MIF), secreted by the embryonic testes, causes regression of the Muellerian structures (the embryonic uterus and fallopian tubes) and preserves the development of the Wolffian structures (the epididymis, vas deferens, and prostate). The predominance of either Muellerian structures or their Wolffian counterparts signals to the investigator the internal phenotypic sex.

In a fetus with testes, the secretion of testosterone and its subsequent conversion to dihydrotestosterone cause two things to happen: the fetal labioscrotal folds fuse to form the scrotum, into which the testes normally descend, and the phallus enlarges into a penis, with the migration of the urethra along the penis so that the opening is at the tip of the glans. In a fetus lacking functional testes, the conversion enzyme, or the hormone receptors, the labioscrotal folds form labia and the fetal phallus becomes a clitoris. These physical changes of the genitals determine the newborn's external *phenotypic sex.* Using the gestalt appearance of the phenotypic features at birth, the birth attendant typically makes the pronouncement "It's a boy!" or "It's a girl!" and this in turn determines the sex of rearing. (In intersex cases, this pronouncement may be delayed as noted below.)

Sex of rearing refers to parents' identification of the child as either a boy or a girl. Studies report that differing maternal (and paternal) behavior patterns for boys and girls begin in the first few days after birth. These continue on in such issues as choice of style in clothes and types of toys. The sex of rearing is determined by the parents' interpretation of the child's anatomic appearance, and the input from the medical personnel around the time of delivery.

Gender differs from sex in that, whereas sex is usually thought of as representing the composite of physical characteristics, gender represents the individual's psychological and emotional identification as either male or female. Stable gender identity is often assumed only as an adult. Transsexed individuals report the identification of the incongruence (between sex and gender) beginning in childhood or adolescence. Hence the division of gender in table 12-1 into that of childhood and that of adulthood.

INTERSEX CONDITIONS

Intersex conditions are those in which an individual's physical development does not follow the standard steps in the pathway from genetic sex to adult gender. The newborn with ambiguous genitalia forms the prototypical case, but not all cases of intersex are recognized at birth because intersexed children may be born with fairly standard-looking genitalia.

The most common cause of intersex is an enzymatic error called congenital adrenal hyperplasia (CAH), which results in a genetic (XX) and gonadally female fetus making substantial amounts of testosterone, which, in turn, virilize (masculinize) the external genitalia. By contrast, XY gonadal dysgenesis occurs when, despite the presence of an apparently normal Y chromosome, the testes fail to develop properly. Most commonly this results in a fibrous band or "streak gonad," which may still have some degree of hormonal activity. Mixed gonadal dysgenesis also usually involves streak gonads; in cases of mixed gonadal dysgenesis, individuals may have a mosaic karyotype, which blends different chromosomal constitutions, such as some XX, some XY, and some XO (where "O" represents an absence of a second sex chromosome).

During prenatal development, individuals with 5-alpha reductase (5-AR) deficiency cannot convert testosterone to the more potent dihydrotestosterone. In spite of being genetically and gonadally male, they are born looking fairly feminine in external genital appearance. By contrast, individuals with androgen insensitivity syndrome (AIS) also have testes and an XY chromosomal pattern, but lack the receptors to respond to androgens. Even within these intersex conditions, the degree of the anomaly can vary; thus complete AIS (CAIS) results in a female external phenotype despite normal male chromosomes and testes, while partial AIS (PAIS) and 5-AR deficiency still permit some degree of virilization concordant with the degree of residual receptor or hormonal activity.

True hermaphrodites are defined as those people with both ovarian and testicular tissue. This can occur as separate gonads, such as a testis on the right and an ovary on the left, or as a mixture of ovarian and testicular elements in each gonad (called ovotestes). These individuals exhibit a wide variety of chromosomal constitutions and a highly variable phenotypic picture internally and externally.

Other conditions may represent a change in the normal sexual developmental pattern but result in less confusion at birth as to the sex.

Micropenis and clitoromegaly are variations in size, as their names suggest. In cases of simple micropenis or clitoromegaly, the presence of other standard anatomic traits usually gives a clear idea of the predominant sex. Klinefelter's syndrome and Turner's syndrome are chromosomal abnormalities in which, respectively, a boy has more than one X chromosome while still having a Y (XXY most commonly) or a girl is missing part or all of her second X chromosome. *Hypospadias*, by definition, occurs in an apparently male child in whom the urethral meatus (exit of the urethra) opens somewhere other than at the tip of the penis, either on the underside of the penis or at its base. The erect penis often is significantly curved as well (chordee).

OLD PARADIGM

Modern medicine began assessing and describing intersexed individuals in increasing numbers in the last century. Victorian experts established a practice of labeling each individual's "true sex" according to the individual's gonadal sex.[2] This process was not easy to apply to ambiguous newborns, nor did its determinations correlate well with gender identity or external phenotypic features in many cases, including, for example, in CAIS.

Because of these shortcomings, many practitioners in the 1920s abandoned the gonadal definition of "true sex" for intersex cases. Beginning in the 1950s, the group at Johns Hopkins University, headed by John Money, championed the "optimum sex of rearing" approach.[3] This approach is based on evaluation of the "ambiguous" newborn as a "psychosocial emergency." The rush to complete the evaluation represents an effort to avoid unnecessary trauma to the family. After all, what is the first question anyone asks the family of a newborn baby?

The emergency evaluation typically includes a urologist (preferably pediatric), a pediatric endocrinologist, and a geneticist.[4] These experts assess the child, determine an "optimum" sex of rearing, and make the child's sex assignment. Sexual function for genetic males and fertility for genetic females are the major considerations. The main basis for the decision revolves around the potential for surgical "reconstruction"; the urologist (who is a surgeon) passes judgment on this potential. If, in a genetic male, there is not a phallus of sufficient size to be easily made into an acceptable penis, then the clinicians prefer a female gender assignment. If the child has ovaries and a uterus, then the physicians see fertility as the primary consideration, and they choose to assign the child to the female gender. If there is pronounced ambiguity, once again most clinicians generally recommend a female gender assignment. This preference for female gender assignments is based on the surgical opinion that it is easier to construct a functional (passive) vagina than a functional (potentially erectile) penis.[5]

The endocrinologist's most critical roles are to evaluate the child for CAH, which could have life-threatening consequences if missed, and to establish the plan for hormone-replacement therapy based on the urologist's plan for operative reconstruction. The geneticist determines the genetic/chromosomal make-up and contributes to the understanding of the underlying anomaly that resulted in the intersex condition. The family is then informed of the medical team's decision about the child's sex assignment and the clinicians' plans for surgically and hormonally bringing the child's appearance in line with the assigned sex.

In most cases, the medical team will recommend that surgical therapy begin early in order to spare parents the trauma of seeing their child as intersexed each time they change the infant's diaper.[6] Further, early surgery is intended to minimize questions and comments by others who may see the child. These surgeries generally include, for children assigned male, attempts to create a "normal" scrotum and to correct any hypospadias. For children assigned female, surgeons remove or reduce in size the "enlarged clitoris" (the "unreconstructable" penis) and, if they deem it necessary, divide the rudimentary scrotum into divided labia. The surgeons may perform vaginoplasties (construction of "vaginas") at highly variable ages, depending on the adults' perception of the child's appearance and the preferences of the surgeons. It is important to note that there is no data that surgery, either early or late, has any positive psychological impact on the parents, let alone the child.

At the time of initial gender assignment, to protect the child's psychosexual development from potentially hurtful comments, physicians have generally counseled families not to discuss any of this with other family members or friends. Further, based on the theory that any doubt may undermine development of a gender identity concordant with the assigned sex of rearing, they also advise the family not to discuss the child's condition with the child. Parents are instructed to make follow-up appointments with the urologist according to the intended and actual operative and post-operative course. The endocrinologist generally sees the child again at the time when puberty should occur, in order to start hormone-replacement therapy. Since the genetic component will have already been evaluated, clinicians consider genetic follow up unnecessary unless the genital abnormalities appear to be part of a larger genetic syndrome with other significant implications for health or development.

PROBLEMS

So, what is wrong with this plan? The recurring voices of many individuals treated in accordance with this paradigm increasingly indicate that it just does not work the way it is supposed to work.[7] These individuals see much of their trauma as generated by the medical care system. Among the problems first and foremost is the lack of true communication. The medical team frequently makes sex assignments with little, if any, involvement of the family—even though they acknowledge that the entire success of the assignment is based on the family's unambiguous rearing of the child as the assigned sex.[8]

The attempts to keep any question of sex or gender from entering into the child's mind result in the recommendation that the child not be told his or her true condition or diagnosis. But as most experienced parents will note, children have a particular knack for recognizing when something is being withheld from them, especially when scars, appearances, and frequent doctor visits document that something about them *is* different. Thus, it may be fallacy to suppose that secrecy as to this difference can be maintained. Again, there are no studies that document the psychological impact of secrecy versus open discussion, and the ethics of such withholding of information has recently been debated.[9]

This silence can create significant feelings of shame.[10] After all, what could be so wrong with a child that his/her own parents won't discuss it with him/her? The child may well feel different, defective, or inadequate. Ultimately, as with most attempts to keep diagnostic/prognostic information from a child (or any patient for that matter), the truth is not as devastating as what the child imagines. The feeling of shame, of somehow having failed, persists and can negatively flavor multiple areas of emotional development.[11]

The actual surgery poses problems as well. Despite efforts to preserve the neurovascular bundle that permits sexual sensation and orgasm, many surgeries to "reconstruct" a "normal sized" clitoris or penis result in decreased sensation and/or function. The approach to surgery is fairly individualized; for example, until recently, there were no data on the range of clitoral size, so surgery has been based on the surgeon's personal perspective of "normal" clitoral size. Even now, although clitoral measurements have been reported in the literature,[12] they fail to appear in such reference works as the *Handbook of Normal Physical Dimensions*.[13] The surgical approach has become more elaborate over time. Clitorectomy (removal of the clitoris) has generally been replaced by clitoral reduction (removing much tissue but attempting to spare the neurovascular bundle) and clitoral recession (burying part of the shaft of the clitoris to make it less visible). However, the evaluation of results of the newer techniques is still subjective and done by the surgeon, typically focusing on short-term cosmetic appearance.[14] The definition of a "successful" surgical result may well differ in the eyes of the surgeon and the eyes of the patient.

In addition, there are many reports of the sex of rearing and the adult gender differing.[15] In at least two,[16] the rearing is reported to have been unambiguously consistent with the infantile sex assignment. These cases cast doubt on the precept that if a child is raised strictly as male or female, then that will remain his or her gender identity. There is considerable support for the theory that there may be a neurobiologic component to many gender identities. Levels of androgens may affect the brain prenatally or immediately postnatally.[17] The what, when, and how of hormonal influences on the sexual differentiation of the brain are just beginning to be understood. Certainly, gender development involves more than the behaviors of the parents in rearing the child.

Finally, this is an age of increasing patients' autonomy. The courts and the public now clearly view medical records as the property of the patient. More and more patients are obtaining and reading their own medical records. For the written record to contradict the information that has been told to the patient is potentially very upsetting and unethical. For the contradiction to be pointed out by third-party inquiries, such as insurance company databases, to whom the records may have been released, is even more upsetting to the patients. Yet these types of problems have happened repeatedly in the case of intersex diagnoses.

Similarly, the right of the individual to determine what happens to his or her body has been increasingly asserted. Patients and families are demanding a voice in the issue of sex assignments and therapies. After all, the child's sex-of-rearing and gender identity are profoundly important to that child's lifelong development and adjustment. Although parents may give consent for surgery, there is increasing movement toward obtaining a child's assent to procedures, particularly those which, like most genital "reconstructive" procedures, are elective from a medical viewpoint. This means delaying surgery until we can take into account the affected individual's determination of his or her own gender.

NEW PARADIGM

That the old treatment methods were not successful is clear from the raised voices of former patients with clear objections to their medical treatment, as well as from recent data.[18] These include objections to the surgeries performed, to the sex-assignment methods, and, perhaps most importantly, to the psychological and emotional treatment (or lack thereof). In response to the identified problems with the methodology described above, a new evaluation and treatment paradigm is emerging.

This new paradigm begins by challenging the idea that the gender assignment of an intersexed newborn must be treated as an emergency. Instead the new paradigm treats sex assignment as urgent, but notes that the only true *medical* emergency in the vast majority of newborns with intersex conditions is the evaluation for congenital adrenal hyperplasia (which can cause a life-threatening metabolic crisis within the first few days or weeks after birth). Otherwise clinicians can take time sufficient to assure a rational and comprehensive evaluation, rather than following the quick rule that males require primarily "adequate" penile size and females require primarily preservation of fertility. While a very few intersexuals argue that it would be preferable to totally withhold gender assignment until the child is old enough to participate,[19] most laypersons (including intersexuals) and professionals still do not see this as feasible in our current society. However, it is increasingly clear that it is more important that the assignment be right than that it be fast. It is also increasingly clear that children can come to recognize their differing gender identity from their infancy-assigned identity without major psychological collapse or psychiatric illness.[20]

Under the new system, the neonatal gender assignment team still includes a urologist, a geneticist, and a pediatric endocrinologist. However, the team now includes the parents. After all, it will be their actions on a daily basis that will behaviorally reinforce or cast doubt on the gender assignment decision. This can be an awkward position for the parents, as they are expected to function within a group of "experts" at the same time that they are grieving the loss of their expected "perfect" child. This is just one reason among many that it becomes very important to include a child psychiatrist with liaison experience or a pediatric psychologist on the decision-making team. These professionals, particularly the psychiatrist who is a physician, have a background in working with children with both chronic and acute medical problems (which the more general child psychologist or social worker usually lacks). Thus they understand the medical decision-making process and can offer the family ongoing support for internal issues (like grief and fear), while at the same time facilitating accurate and complete communication between the medical members of the decision-making team and the parents. This role is often necessary to facilitate the family's very central role in the gender assignment decision. In addition, referral to a support group (either diagnosis-specific or more general, such as the Intersex Society of North America) can be vastly reassuring. These groups provide both empathy and advice based on their experience with the condition and the medical care system.

Early uro-genital surgery should be strictly limited to that necessary to preserve the child's health,[21] that is, primarily those surgeries necessary to establish normal urinary tract function and to correct conditions that could cause recurrent infections or other damaging physical effects. Gonadectomy (removal of the gonads) should be restricted to those cases where dysgenic (maldeveloped) gonads are present in an individual with Y chromosomal material, particularly if the karyotype is abnormal (other than 46 XY or 47 XXY). Gonadoblastoma (cancer of the gonads) has been seen in such infants as young as 14 months of age.[22] Delaying removal of the gonads in other cases permits the maximum chance for fertility (a chance that increases every year with progress made in reproductive technologies) and for endogenous (physiological) production of hormones for puberty and through adulthood.

Further, consistent with the increasing emphasis on patient-centered medicine, leaving the gonads allows the patient to retain vital body parts until her or she is mature enough to participate in the medical decision-making process. While an older child or early adolescent may not be able to fully understand all of the medical reasoning and options, delay at least permits the child to help identify his/her own gender—a fact that should determine the nature of the reconstructions to be undertaken. Holmes and colleagues have described such use of surgery to reinforce adolescent gender identification, including a case where an adolescent's gender identity contradicted the sex of rearing.[23] By contrast, a recent referral involved a child diagnosed as a true hermaphrodite with a female sex assignment referred by her pediatric psychologist. Her endocrinologist wanted to use estrogen therapy early to quiet the child's feelings of perhaps being male. But such an attempt to deny the child's sense of identity and suppress the gender confusion would seem to risk greater gender confusion and conflict as an adult, similar to that experienced by transsexuals. In addition, there is no data that feminizing hormones affect the evolution of gender identity. We recommended delaying hormone therapy until the child has a chance, with the help of her psychologist, to come to some decision about her gender identity.

It follows that if the child is to become a part of the decision-making team as he or she matures, then consistently open and accurate communication with the child regarding his or her condition and medical/surgical history is critical. Ongoing involvement with several members of the treatment team, such as the pediatric endocrinologist and urologist, can assure this. The continued involvement of the pediatric psychologist or psychiatrist can help the family answer the child's questions in honest and age-appropriate ways and can help facilitate open and clear communication between the child, the family, and the medical team. Many families are so devastated during the initial phases of their child's evaluation and treatment that they may not fully comprehend and absorb the information presented to them. For example, another recent referral involved a family with a daughter, now 13 years old, with complete androgen insensitivity syndrome. Despite two visits with the endocrinologist and a genetics clinic visit in the first year of life when the diagnosis was made, at present the family only understood that their daughter had had abnormal gonads and that she would not be able to have babies. Ongoing involvement with the psychiatrist or psychologist could have facilitated more effective communication and education for both the parents and the child (and perhaps a referral to the AIS support groups), resulting in less trauma as this girl enters adolescence, with its self-examination and identity exploration.

As we have seen, the new paradigm takes into account the input of family and child and responds to the progress made in the medical and surgical fields. The process must involve ongoing and recurrent re-evaluations and caution where irreversible treatments are concerned. Hormonal therapy should be reserved until the patient is able to define his or her own gender identity, and should be consistent with this identity, regardless of the gender of rearing. Conducting periodic but regular standardized gender assessment schedules with the patient and the parents may provide information to aid in this process.[24] Surgical genitoplasty (such as that described in the opening case history) should not be performed until the patient can fully consent to the procedure. Further, consent information should include risks such as reduced sexual sensation, less than perfect cosmetic results, and possible interference with sexual function.

In order to support the new approach, it is important that the medical team and family understand the degree of normal variation in genital anatomy and the number of unanswered questions where gender development is concerned. They must also be aware that, despite the best efforts of all concerned, a person may identify with a different gender than that of rearing, as non-heterosexual, or (rarely) as non-gendered.[25] Acceptance of this and of the individual can be facilitated by the mental health provider, and may be aided by the voice of experience represented by appropriate support groups.

This new paradigm is not without its own complexities and potential problems. First, the emergence of this protocol is, in large part, the result of a relatively small number of very vocal former patients and of a pilot study of six adolescents sex-reassigned at birth.[26] These individuals are obviously upset with the surgeries that have been performed on them, as well at the lack of communication and support they have received both from the medical team and from their families. As we shift to the new paradigm, it would be reassuring if there were a body of data gleaned from individuals with ambiguous genitalia who had not undergone surgery to tell us that they had not suffered additional psychological or emotional problems because of the delay in or lack of surgical repair. Some such voices are beginning to be heard,[27] but there are also a few who wish they had had surgery as young children.[28]

Similarly, there is little data about whether families can provide children with ambiguous physical appearances unambiguous rearing, or whether they can accept change in gender status when it occurs. (For that matter, it is assumed such unambiguous rearing occurs after early cosmetic genital surgery, but data to support this is lacking.) The question of the interaction with peers is also critical; the middle school/junior high years often bring pejorative teasing about any perceived differences. Again, data from intersex individuals who underwent early, late, or no surgical "repair" will be critical to our understanding of these issues.

DISCUSSION

When one chooses to adopt a new treatment in medicine, it is usually based on data that the new protocol provides superior results in the majority of patients. In the case of treatment of intersex children, such studies have not been performed, although at least two authors have called for such data collection in the process of defending the status quo.[29] The first obstacle is that, to fully assess the impact of each approach, one would have to wait for the full maturity of the individuals to get an accurate picture of any physical, psychological, or emotional morbidity associated with each type of treatment. Thus a study started today would need to follow each individual for 30 or more years, a logistically unfeasible duration. In addition, each manifestation of intersex is somewhat different and may depend upon complex sociocultural factors. An argument could be made for separate studies for each condition with controls for socio-cultural context.

In order to begin addressing this area, one of the authors (WGR) is embarking on a five-year study assessing longitudinally a series of patients with a homogeneous diagnosis who have been sex-reassigned at birth. Appropriate controls for each target subject have been selected for illness/surgical conditions, socioeconomic status, peer-age, and both genders. Children, adolescents, and young adults will be chosen, providing a fairly full life picture through age 30. Additional intersex conditions will be added separately as the study progresses.

As with many clinical paradigm shifts, in the absence of data, adherents of each protocol become increasingly dogmatic that their preferred approach is better for the patient, and that it would be unethical to subject the patient to the other, "less acceptable" treatment. Individual clinicians' attachments to specific treatment regimes result in the ongoing polarization of paradigms. While the new intersex paradigm is consistent with the evolving "patient-centered" approach to medical care, under it there remains a possibility of doing harm to the patient by delaying medical and surgical intervention. Indeed, the surgical literature on intersex argues that even repeated genital surgeries are less traumatic to the emotional development of a child than to be, for example, raised as a girl without a vagina.[30] Such arguments are often prefaced by words such as "in our experience," yet methodologically sound data do not exist.

Money has presented some data that having a child with ambiguous genitalia causes parental stress,[31] but support for the second part of the hypothesis, that the stress on parent (and presumably also child) is alleviated by surgical correction, is entirely absent. In fact, the approach to the family is almost entirely absent from major articles on the approach to the intersex infant; typically parents leave all decisions in the hands of the physicians. The increased mental health participation, the more effective communication, and the new study being initiated should allow better assessment of the new paradigm and its effects on patients and families.

Surgical follow-up data have reflected the surgeons', and not the patients', determinations of "acceptable," "adequate," "cosmetic," and "functional" outcomes. Numerous unhappy patients attest to the failure of surgical treatment. Thus the new paradigm is cast in the mold of one of the oldest medical axioms: "First do no harm." The new paradigm involves patient and family in both the early decision-making process and the long-term evaluation. While the rush to surgery is based on the attempt to prevent trauma, an admirable goal, data that it furthers this goal are lacking. Similarly, arguments that the newest surgical techniques give dramatically improved results also are being accepted without follow-up evaluation. Two recent articles document that when evaluation was performed on "new procedures" that had gained significant popularity, each new procedure's results were actually at the same level or worse that previous techniques.[32]

It is interesting to note that ambiguous genitalia are essentially the only congenital anomalies viewed as a surgical emergency for cosmetic reasons. This mirrors the emphasis on gender within our society yet fails to address the unknowns in the ever more complex picture of bio-psychosocial determinants of gender-identity development. In view of the absence of clear scientific or empirical data to support current interventive strategies, it appears to be most reasonable to avoid early irreversible interventions and to allow patients the central role in determining what will happen to their bodies.

ACKNOWLEDGMENT

This chapter first appeared in *The Journal of Clinical Ethics* 9, no. 4 (Winter 1998); © 1998 by *The Journal of Clinical Ethics*; used with permission.

NOTES

1. A.D. Dreger, "A History of Intersexuality: From the Age of Gonads to the Age of Consent," chapter 1 of this volume; A.D. Dreger, *Hermaphrodites and the Medical Invention of Sex* (Cambridge, Mass.: Harvard Press, 1998), 139-66.

2. Ibid.

3. J. Money, J.G. Hampson, and J.L. Hampson, "Hermaphroditism: Recommendations Concerning Assignment of Sex, Change of Sex, and Psychologic Management," *Bulletin of the Johns Hopkins Hospital* 97 (1955): 284-300; J. Money, J.G. Hampson, and J.L. Hampson, "An Examination of Some Basic Sexual Concepts: The Evidence of Human Hermaphroditism," *Bulletin of the Johns Hopkins Hospital* 97 (1955): 301-19; H.F.L. Meyer-Bahlburg, "Gender Assignment in Intersexuality," *Journal of Psychology & Human Sexuality* 10, no. 2 (1998): 1-21.

4. M.O. Savage, "Ambiguous Genitalia, Small Genitalia and Undescended

Testes," *Clinics in Endocrinology and Metabolism* 11, no. 1 (1982): 127-58; R.A. Pagon, "Diagnostic Approach to the Newborn with Ambiguous Genitalia," *Pediatric Clinics of North America* 34, no. 4 (1987): 1019-31.

5. Z. Krstic et al., "Surgical Treatment of Intersex Disorders," *Journal of Pediatric Surgery* 30, no. 9 (1995): 1273-81. For a criticism of this treatment, see A.D. Dreger, " 'Ambiguous Sex'—Or Ambivalent Medicine? Ethical Issues in the Treatment of Intersexuality," *Hastings Center Report* 28, no. 3 (May-June 1998): 24-35.

6. Meyer-Bahlburg, "Gender Assignment in Intersexuality," see note 3 above.

7. For representative narration of this issue, see *Hermaphrodites Speak!* a video publication of the Intersex Society of North America (C. Chase, *Hermaphrodites Speak!* Intersex Society of North America, 26 minutes, 1997, video-cassette. Copies may be obtained from ISNA, PO Box 31791, San Francisco, Calif. 94131; website < www.isna.org >); the website "Intersex Voices" website < http://www.qis.net/ ~ triea >, (particularly the "Real People" and "Other Voices" sections); and multiple articles in "Special Issue on Intersexuality," *Chrysalis: The Journal of Transgressive Gender Identities* 2, no. 5 (Fall 1997/Winter 1998).

8. C.H. Meyers-Seifer and N.J. Charest, "Diagnosis and Management of Patients with Ambiguous Genitalia," *Seminars in Perinatology* 16, no. 5 (1992): 332-39.

9. A. Natarajan, "Medical Ethics and Truth Telling in the Case of Androgen Insensitivity Syndrome," *Canadian Medical Association Journal* 154, no. 4 (1996): 568-70; and letters in response (multiple authors), "Sex, Lies and the Androgen Insensitivity Syndrome," *Canadian Medical Association Journal* 154, no. 12 (1996): 1829-33.

10. In this volume: S.A. Groveman, "The Hanukkah Bush," chapter 2; S.E. Preves, "For the Sake of the Children: Destigmatizing Intersexuality," chapter 4; M. Coventry, "Finding the Words," chapter 5; H. Devore, "Growing Up in the Surgical Maelstrom," chapter 6; D. Cameron, "Caught Between: An Essay on Intersexuality," chapter 8; A. Moreno, "In Amerika They Call Us Hermaphrodites," chapter 13; and H. Walcutt, "Time for a Change," chapter 19. Also, *Hermaphrodites Speak*, see note 7 above; the website "Intersex Voices" (particularly the "Real People" and "Other Voices" sections), see note 7 above; and multiple articles in the "Special Issue on Intersexuality," in *Chrysalis*, see note 7 above.

11. Ibid.

12. K. Sane and O.H. Pescovitz, "The Clitoral Index: A Determination of Size in Normal Girls and in Girls with Abnormal Sexual Development," *Journal of Pediatrics* 120, no. 2 (1992): 264-66; B.S. Verkauf, J. von Thron, and W. O'Brien, "Clitoral Size in Normal Women," *Obstetrics & Gynecology* 80, no. 1 (1992): 41-44; A. Litwin, I. Aitkin, and P. Merlob, "Clitoral Length Assessment in Newborn Infants of 30 to 41 Weeks Gestational Age," *European Journal of Obstetrics & Gynecology and Reproductive Biology* 38 (1990): 209-12; S.E. Oberfield

et al., "Clitoral Size in Full-Term Infants," *American Journal of Perinatology* 6 (1989): 453-54.

13. J.G. Hall, U.G. Frosster-Iskenius, and J.E. Allanson, *Handbook of Normal Physical Measurements* (Oxford, England: Oxford University Press, 1989).

14. T.P.V.M. de Jong and T.M.L. Boemers, "Neonatal Management of Female Intersex by Clitorovaginoplasty," *Journal of Urology* 154 (1995): 830-32.

15. W.G. Reiner, "Case Study: Sex Reassignment in a Teenage Girl," *Journal of the American Academy of Child and Adolescent Psychiatry* 35, no. 6 (1996): 799-803; S.A.V. Holmes et al., "Surgical Reinforcement of Gender Identity in Adolescent Intersex Patients," *Urologia Internationalis* 48 (1992): 430-33; M. Diamond and J.K. Sigmundson, "Sex Reassignment at Birth: Long-Term Review and Clinical Implications," *Archives of Pediatric and Adolescent Medicine* 151 (1997): 298-304.

16. W.G. Reiner, "Case Study: Sex Reassignment in a Teenage Girl," *Journal of the American Academy of Child and Adolescent Psychiatry* 35, no. 6 (1996): 799-803; Diamond and Sigmundson, "Sex Reassignment at Birth," see note 15 above.

17. R.A. Gorski, "Sexual Differentiation of the Endocrine Brain and Its Control," in *Brain Endocrinology*, 2d ed., ed. M. Motta (New York: Raven, 1991); M. Diamond, T. Binstock, and J.V. Kohl, "From Fertilization to Adult Sexual Behavior," *Hormones and Behavior* 30 (1996): 333-53.

18. W.G. Reiner, "To Be Male or Female—That is the Question," *Archives of Pediatric and Adolescent Medicine* 151 (1997): 224-25; W.G. Reiner, unpublished data. Readers may contact W.G. Reiner at <wreiner@jhmi.edu> for more information.

19. E. Nevada, "Lucky to Have Escaped Genital Surgery," *Hermaphrodites with Attitude* (electronic newsletter of ISNA, on website <www.isna.org>) (1997).

20. Ibid.; W.G. Reiner, unpublished data (contact W.G. Reiner at <wreiner@jhmi.edu> for a discussion of the data).

21. Intersex Society of North America, "Recommendations for Treatment of Intersex Infants and Children", published on the ISNA website <http://www.isna.org/recommendations.htm>; M. Diamond and H.K. Sigmundson, "Management of Intersexuality," *Archives of Pediatric and Adolescent Medicine* 151 (1997): 1046-50.

22. B.E. Wilson, "Down-Turner Blend—An Expansion of Phenotypic Expression," (unpublished manuscript, 1998). Readers may contact B.E. Wilson at <wilsonbb@pilot.msu.edu>.

23. Holmes et al., "Surgical Reinforcement of Gender Identity," see note 15 above.

24. J.E. Bates, P.M. Bentler, and S.K. Thompson, "Gender Deviant Boys Compared With Normal and Clinical Control Boys," *Journal of Abnormal Child Psychology* 7, no. 3 (1979): 243-59; J.E. Bates, P.M. Bentler, and S.K. Thompson, "Measurement of Deviant Gender Development in Boys," *Child Development*

44, no. 3 (1973): 591-98; H.F.L. Meyer-Bahlburg, J.F. Feldman, and A.A. Ehrhardt, "Questionnaire for the Assessment of Atypical Gender Role Behavior: A Methodological Study," *Journal of the American Academy of Child and Adolescent Psychiatry* 24, no. 6 (1985): 695-701; M. Paluszny et al., "Gender Identity and Its Measurement in Children," *Comprehensive Psychiatry* 14, no. 3 (1973): 281-90.

25. R.J. Stoller, "The Hermaphroditic Identity of Hermaphrodites," *Journal of Nervous and Mental Disorders* 139 (1964): 453-57.

26. For representative narration of this issue, see *Hermaphrodites Speak!* see note 7 above; the website "Intersex Voices," see note 7 above; and multiple articles in the "Special Issue on Intersexuality" in *Chrysalis,* see note 7 above; and W.G. Reiner, unpublished data, see note 18 above.

27. Nevada, "Lucky," see note 19 above; in this volume, see Kim, "As Is," chapter 9; H. Hawbecker, "Who Did This to You?" chapter 11.

28. Diane [last name withheld], "A Retrospective Review of a Male Pseudo-Hermaphrodite's Long Road to Recovery," electronic publication, website "Intersex Voices," the "Real People" section, see note 7 above.

29. Meyer-Bahlburg, "Gender Assignment in Intersexuality," see note 3 above; D. Sandberg, "A Call for Clinical Research," *Hermaphrodites with Attitude* (electronic newsletter of ISNA, on website < www.isna.org >) (Fall-Winter 1995-1996).

30. W.H. Hendren and A. Atala, "Use of Bowel for Vaginal Reconstruction," *Journal of Urology* 152 (1994): 752-55.

31. Money, Hampson, and Hampson, "Hermaphroditism: Recommendations Concerning Assignment of Sex, Change of Sex, and Psychologic Management," see note 3 above.

32. F.T. Vertosick, "First Do No Harm," *Discover* 19, no. 7 (1998): 106-11; J.A. Talcott et al., "Patient-Reported Impotence and Incontinence after Nerve-Sparing Radical Prostatectomy," *Journal of the National Cancer Institute* 89, no. 15 (1997): 1117-23.

13

In Amerika They Call Us Hermaphrodites

Angela Moreno

> *doctors have come from distant cities*
> *just to see me—stand over my bed*
> *disbelieving what they're seeing*
> *they say I must be one of the wonders*
> *of god's own creation*
> —Natalie Merchant, "Wonder,"
> from the album *Tiger Lily*

There was never any reason to suspect anything strange. I appeared female when I was born in 1972, and I was assigned and raised as a girl.

When I was 12, I started to notice that my clitoris (that wonderful location of pleasure for which I had no name but to which I had grown quite attached) had grown more prominent. At least, that's how I perceived it. I can't remember whether I thought anything about it; I just remember that I began to notice it. I'm sure that it was at least three months after I had taken note that my mother caught a glimpse of me as I bathed one day after returning from the dance studio. She tried very hard not to let on how alarmed she was, but of course a 12-year-old girlchild just senses these things. When the pediatrician examined me the next day she was also obviously alarmed. She referred me to a female pediatric endocrinologist at the University of Illinois College of Medicine, Peoria.

Exactly one month later, I was admitted to Children's Memorial Hospital in Chicago for surgery. They told me a little bit about the part where they were going to "remove my ovaries" because they suspected cancer or something like that. They didn't mention the part where they were going to slice off my clitoris. All of it. I guess the doctors assumed I was as horrified by my outsized clit as they were, and there was no need to discuss it with me. After a week's recovery in the hospital, we all went home and barely ever spoke of it again.

As for the assertion that doctors now consistently provide sophisticated counseling for the intersexed child and family, my experience does not reflect that good intention. First of all, my doctors made a traumatizing hospitalization even more traumatizing by putting me on show for parades of earnest young residents with "you're-a-freak-but-we're-compassionate" grins on their faces. This, all without nurses or my parents anywhere around. Second, I know now from my parents that the pediatric endocrinologists repeatedly advised them that I did not need to know the truth. They told my parents some horror story about a girl like me who had peeked at her file once while the doctor was out of the room and then killed herself. My mother asked the doctors specifically if they thought I would benefit from any type of counseling. They discouraged her from pursuing it. That's what passed for emotional support among the Children's Memorial Hospital intersex specialist team in Chicago in 1985.

Now 24, I've spent the last 10 years in a haze of disordered eating and occasional depression. My struggle with bulimia has been an all-consuming although mostly secret part of my life, and I now believe it represents my attempts to express the fear, shame, rage, and intense body-hatred that I have felt as a result of the—until now—unspeakable assault that I experienced under the guise of medical treatment.

I do have some clitoral sensation. I sometimes masturbate and I do have an experience that I call orgasm—some faint muscular contractions. But response is unreliable, and nothing like the tremendous sensitivity and wonderful juicy orgasms I had before the clitoral surgery. I would say that the clitoral recession and vaginoplasty decreased my responsiveness by a factor of five or 10.

Four months ago, I finally got some of my medical records from Children's Memorial Hospital, in Chicago. They are shocking. The surgeon who removed my clitoris summarized the outcome as "tolerated well."

I hadn't made much sense of these records until a recent visit to my gynecologist, at Barnes Hospital in St. Louis. I was referred to her three years ago, by the University of Illinois pediatric endocrinologist, to determine whether I would "need" the vaginoplasty. This was all news to me as I had never been informed that I would ever need more surgery. As it turned out, my gynecologist concluded that I had a sufficient vagina and she recommended only pressure dilation.

Anyway, just about a month ago I visited the gynecologist for my routine annual physical—she's the only doctor I ever see. This time, when she asked what kinds of questions I had, I pulled out my records and asked her to review them with me. She actually spent over an hour with me explaining some of my records to me. One phrase that stuck in my head was "Androgen Insensitivity Syndrome." I left that day still in a fog, but a little more confident that at least someone had taken my questions seriously.

Then, just under a week ago, I received a package by mail from a friend in whom I had confided some very sketchy details about my surgery. Natalie Angier's article about ISNA[1] and the Winter 1995-1996 issue of ISNA's newsletter, *Hermaphrodites with Attitude,* had crossed her desk, and she realized that this might be related to my situation. In fact she was absolutely right. I couldn't believe it as I sat there reading stories that I could have written. After reading these articles and others that I located at the ISNA website,[2] I now suspect that I have Partial Androgen Insensitivity Syndrome. The medical team lied to me about removing my ovaries; they actually removed my testes. I know from my records that I have a 46 XY karyotype.

I am horrified by what has been done to me and by the conspiracy of silence and lies. I am filled with grief and rage, but also relief finally to believe that maybe I am not the only one. My doctor told me more than once that I wasn't the only one, but I never got to meet any of them. I'm full of anticipation, fear, and craziness at the thought that, through ISNA, I may finally be able to speak with and meet others who share these experiences.

ACKNOWLEDGMENT

This chapter first appeared in *Chrysalis: The Journal of Transgressive Gender Identities* 2, no. 5 (Fall 1997/Winter 1998); © 1998 by Angela Moreno; used with permission.

NOTES

1. N. Angier, "Intersexual Healing," *New York Times,* Week in Review, 4 February 1996.
2. The Intersex Society of North America website is <www.isna.org>.

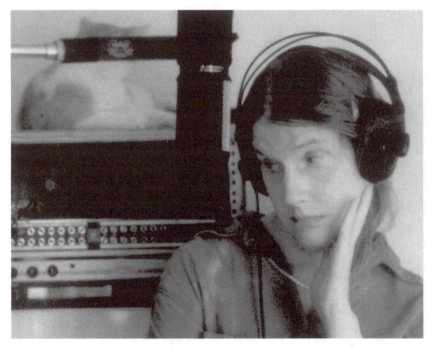

Kiira Triea

14

Power, Orgasm, and the Psychohormonal Research Unit

Kiira Triea

I've wondered why researchers at Johns Hopkins were so concerned with the genitals of a barely teenaged hermaphrodite from a family of absolutely no standing or financial resources. My experience at the PRU [Psychohormonal Research Unit] leads me to believe that a need to express and preserve androcentric control is at the root of the medical-industrial complex's fascination with my (our) genitals. The amount of medical resources that were brought to bear against a 14-year-old intersexed kid are pretty amazing, considering that life-saving surgery and treatments are routinely denied people at Hopkins. Why all the unsolicited attention?

Doctors act as enforcers of genital and behavioral conformity for the Penis Club. As high priests of the biological technocracy, and as privileged possessors of "secret" knowledge, they wield their power to ensure that only owners of a medically approved, "viable" penis are granted membership in the Penis Club. All others are by default granted membership in the Vagina Club. The penis does need to be "viable," as its purpose is not seen as being for pleasurable gratification, but as the mechanism by which members of the Vagina Club are penetrated. Intersexed neonates who have no clearly defined membership qualifications for either club are modified at Hopkins to become members of the Vagina Club. The fact that I was older meant that they couldn't dismiss my interests in the matter as casually as they do with neonates. The fact that I was already verbal required them to tread with a little more care in their quest to neutralize my hermaphrodite genitals.

Hopkins doctors view themselves as compassionate, helpful people who save lives and alleviate suffering. They assumed that since I was raised as a boy, I must want to become a member of the Penis Club. They attempted to utilize technical means to alleviate my suffering as a "defective male." That was the first gender label that they assigned to me. When I first arrived at the PRU, I was evaluated by John Money. He assumed that I had a male gender and, being 14 years old, knew the "facts of life." He asked me if I wanted to fuck someone or if I wanted to be fucked by someone else. Since I didn't completely understand what he was talking about, he showed me a pornographic movie. I first learned the mechanics of penetrative intercourse from this movie, in which a guy with an immense penis had rough, almost violent, penetrative sex with a woman. Money had drawn another blank, as the movie did nothing but frighten me. This technique probably would have worked if I'd been shown a movie that portrayed kissing, hugging, and soft affection. But Money and Hopkins do not postulate a soft world. Their world is the hard, sex-dipoled landscape of power and domination, peopled with those fortunate denizens who are able to fuck others and those who are equipped only to be fucked.

Like earthlings faced with the arrival of some sensitive and mysterious alien, the PRU psych squads continued their attempts to divine the hermaphrodite creature's "true sex." Not having the sensitivity or intelligence to obtain this information by asking, they decided to inject me with testosterone and observe the results. "Put the electrodes here, the hermaphrodite runs over there. Put the electrodes there, the hermaphrodite runs over here." My reaction to testosterone was considered a litmus test for my eligibility for the Penis Club, and it was a test that I failed completely. At this point they reconsidered their labeling of my gender. Money now decided that I was a "failed male," i.e., female. My "true sex" had been discovered. Like shards of genetic pottery scattered amid the ruins of my childhood, my femaleness manifested in my desire to keep my body, my soft skin and shape and voice, as they were. They shifted gears; now they worked to prepare me for initiation into the Vagina Club.

I go blank when people tell me that "in other cultures, intersexed people were respected as Shamans." This knowledge was of absolutely no value to me at all when I was 14 and faced with either hormonal mutation and surgery or vaginoplasty. But there must be some truth in it, because I can think of no other reason why they would invest so much energy in my genitals. They must have been profoundly awed by my genitals! Since they were different from normal genitals, they must be more powerful! Since I had declined membership ("failed") as a Penis Club initiate, it was of paramount importance to make me a member of the Vagina Club as soon as possible. There was no other alternative.

As a member of the Vagina Club I was treated differently at the PRU. Money no longer talked to me of fucking and being fucked. People called me "sweetheart" or "honey," and tried to talk with me of boy-friends and perhaps even marriage. Money told me a story about another hermaphrodite who had a vaginoplasty and whose boyfriend had even visited her in the hospital. I don't remember hearing the words "orgasm" or "lesbian" the entire time I was there, over three years.

I first had an orgasm four years ago, during what I call The Awaken-ing, in which I became fully aware of my life and the implications of being intersexed. I seriously doubt that Dr. Howard Jones, who per-formed genital surgery on me, paid any consideration at all to that func-tion. I have no clitoris at all; whatever was there before seems to have been relocated, perhaps entered into the witness protection program and now living in Arizona. Jones seems to have taken care, though, to ensure that I was able to be penetrated, as my "vagina" seems to be deep enough to allow for that. Part of my left upper arm was pressed into genital duty here, which bothered me greatly when I came out of surgery. I wish I'd been consulted or at least informed. Of course, why would I need to be informed? The objective was to make the hermaphrodite fuckable.

I have spent the last 23 years crawling free of the wreckage of the impact of my anatomy and biology with the PRU. In the last four years I have managed to get back some of my carry-on baggage: I have become accepting of my intersexuality, orgasmic and sexual, relatively stable, and I have an awareness of myself as a valuable and unique person, an intersexed person who is feminine. I actually think I've done pretty well, considering the technological big guns that were brought to bear on me at the PRU. I've come to the conclusion that my genital grigri must be very strong indeed, a mojo so "viable" and enduring that it protected me from the death they envisioned. Perhaps I should follow my clitoris out to Arizona and become the founder of The Church of the Resurrected Climax. I think, though, that I will stick around, where me and my Magical Snatch can stir up some really troublesome voodoo.

ACKNOWLEDGMENTS

The author works with the Coalition for Intersex Support Activism and Education to provide peer support to intersexual persons: < http:// www.sonic.net/ ~ cisae >.

This chapter first appeared in *Chrysalis: The Journal of Transgressive Gender Identities* 2, no. 5 (Fall 1997/Winter 1998); © 1998 by Kiira Triea; used with permission.

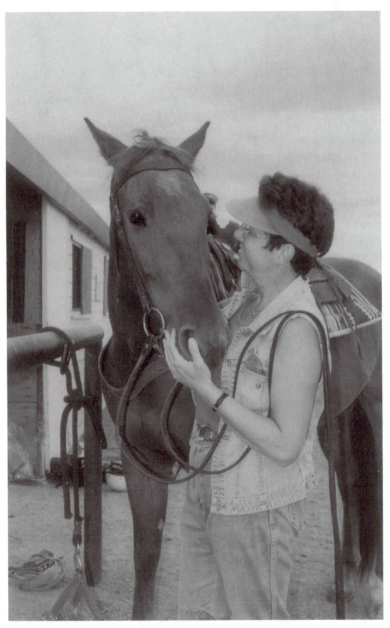

Cheryl Chase

15

Surgical Progress Is Not the Answer to Intersexuality

Cheryl Chase

> *Surgery's* better *now! We're* rapidly *advancing!*
> —Kenneth Glassberg, MD, in an interview about
> intersex surgeries on *Dateline NBC* in 1997

The traditional model of medical treatment of intersexuality has been roundly challenged on ethical and empirical grounds.[1] While they have yet to respond to the ethical challenges, many holdouts for the traditional model insist that criticisms of former patients are irrelevant because "surgery is better now." Practically, there is no evidence to indicate that children operated on with current techniques will have better long-term outcomes than those operated on 10 or more years ago. What is more important, poor surgical outcomes are not the only—or even the primary—reason former patients feel harmed. The primary source of harm described by former patients is not surgery per se, but the underlying attitude that intersexuality is so shameful that it must be erased before the child can have any say in what will be done to his or her body. Early surgery is one means by which that message is conveyed to parents and to intersexed children.[2]

As the director of one of the most visible of the peer support/patient advocacy groups, I have been privileged to communicate with nearly 400 intersexed people and family members. I have seen firsthand hundreds of cases in which well-intentioned but misguided medicine has compounded, rather than alleviated, the difficulties of being born intersexed.[3] Some of this material is available on the internet (see www.isna.org).

Let me say outright that I believe that intersexed children should be labeled male or female,[4] that they should be provided with surgeries or drugs necessary for their *physical* health and well-being, and that for most families intersexuality is and will remain a painful issue. My primary concern is to make the world a safer place for intersexuals and their families. Enlightened doctors will have an important role in this endeavor. Intersexuals old enough to make *informed decisions* should have access to cosmetic surgeries.

A SURGICAL WORLD-VIEW

Surgery is good at removing structures, like infected appendices or localized tumors; it is much less useful for creating structures. When surgeons quip that they prefer to assign intersexed infants female rather than male because "you can dig a hole [that is, a vagina], but you can't build a pole [that is, a penis],"[5] they are acknowledging that theirs is essentially an obliterative, rather than a constructive, art (as well as revealing the crudest imaginable disregard for the complexities of female sexuality).[6]

When genital surgery is performed on an infant, the impact on sexual function cannot be evaluated until sexual maturity, many years later—but these follow-up studies have not been done.[7] For example, although the clitoroplasty technique used on large clitorises in intersex infants was first published over three decades ago, no long-term studies of its impact on sexual function have been done.[8] Surgeons concede that they do not know what impact these surgeries have on intersex children's future sexual function. Johns Hopkins University surgeon John Gearhart says, "We won't know until later whether these patients will be normal and sexually active. We cannot say that they will have orgasms when they are older."[9] A reporter covering a demonstration by former patients who had been sexually mutilated by "reconstructive" surgery related: "As for what happens 21 years later, Robert Jeffs [a colleague of Gearhart] says he has no way of knowing. 'Is this going to be one that's satisfied or one that's out on the street [protesting]? I don't know.' "[10]

In spite of a complete lack of data, many clinicians simply claim that surgeries do in fact preserve sexual function. In the pamphlet, *Becoming a Boy or a Girl,* George Szasz tells parents who are asked to give consent for surgery on their intersexed child that "Female external genitalia will be constructed and reconstructed in a series of operations. A clitoris of appropriate size will be formed from the undeveloped 'penis.' The clitoris has normal sensation."[11] One author even elevated the article of faith, "without loss of sensitivity," into the title of his report,[12] and the accompanying commentary by Milton Edgerton[13] enthused, "For over 40 years, some form of clitorectomy or clitoroplasty has been used to treat little girls with adrenogenital syndrome. The only indication for performing this surgery has been to improve the body image of these children so that they feel 'more normal.' . . . *Not one has complained of loss of sensation even when the entire clitoris was removed* [emphasis in original]."[14] I wrote to complain to Edgerton about loss of sensation and absence of orgasmic response in myself and other intersexed women. He wrote back to acknowledge that even a tiny incision could damage sexual function.[15] Like other clinicians contacted by intersex patients mutilated by genital surgeries, he has not publicly corrected his assertion that genital surgery preserves sexual function. And, as Robert Crouch discusses in this volume, the silence and secrecy of the traditional medical model render former patients voiceless.[16] I believe that if Edgerton had never previously heard a complaint from a former patient, it is not because none has lost genital sensation, but because all were too filled with shame and rage to confront him.

Only careful follow-up data, not surgeons' faith, can show that a new technique is actually better than an old one. For example, until recently surgeons believed that "nerve-sparing" prostate surgery preserved sexual function in most men treated for cancer. Follow-up study, however, now reveals that "nerve sparing" surgery is just about as destructive of sexual function as the traditional surgery.[17] These sorts of results ought to be in the forefront of our thinking when considering claims that current "nerve-sparing" genital surgeries are vastly improved over any surgery performed during infancy or adolescence on an intersex person now old enough to voice a complaint.

Now that some intersexuals are finding a voice with which to complain, a new argument for discounting us has appeared. Gearhart and colleagues measured pudendal nerve latencies during clitoroplasty surgeries and claimed that these electrical measurements, absent any investigation of the girl's actual experience of genital sensation, provided evidence that when grown she would enjoy good sexual function. The authors minimized the importance of a critical letter documenting identical nerve latency in a clitorectomized woman with no orgasmic response with a *non sequitur:* "In fact, some women who have never had surgery are anorgasmic."[18] Coincidental anorgasmia is an unlikely explanation, however, as many intersexed women, including those documented in the letter, are primarily sexual with women. In contrast to heterosexual women, women with extensive homosexual experience who have not had clitoral surgery are infrequently inorgasmic. Kinsey's data reports that 17 percent of married women with five years of coital experience are anorgasmic, and that large numbers achieve orgasm only rarely. Of those women in his sample with extensive homosexual experience, none were anorgasmic, and four-fifths were orgasmic in most of their sexual contacts.[19] Intersexed women with a history of clitoral surgery who have extensive sexual experience with women and are inorgasmic can be fairly certain that the surgery is the cause.

How can surgeons justify the continued practice of surgery with demonstrated risks and no demonstrated benefits? A number of surgeons have expressed—in conversation and in private correspondence, though not in professional publications—the conviction that *any* surgical intervention, no matter how damaging to sexual function or how poor the cosmetic result, is better than leaving an intersexed child unaltered. One woman, searching for help to restore sensation destroyed by a clitorectomy, approached Judson Randolph, a well-known surgeon specializing in clitoroplasty. He told her that clitorectomy had been "all surgeons had to offer" when she was a child.[20] In another case, a man who had been mutilated by over a dozen genital reconstruction surgeries during childhood sought a minor surgery to smooth his surgically constructed penile urethra, which was causing debilitating urinary tract infections. The surgeon, at his own initiative and contrary to the expressed wishes of the anesthetized patient, performed a complete penile reconstruction, which left the man much worse off and motivated him to initiate a lawsuit. A surgeon recruited as an expert witness for the defense remarked that intersexuality was so rare and tragic that "any cutting, no matter how incompetently executed, is a kindness."[21] Again, one of the best-known pediatric endocrinologists in the field recently remarked in conversation that he had never in his career seen a good cosmetic result in intersex genital reconstructions, but "what can you do? The parents demand it."[22]

CATCH-22

Kipnis and Diamond discuss the "epistemological black hole" that precludes follow up of intersex surgeries: the purpose of surgery is to hide intersexuality; therefore, intersexuals must be lied to about their histories and surgeries,[23] and thus follow up cannot be done because the patients would learn the truth.[24] Use of the claim, "surgery is better now," is a strategy for silencing intersexed adults:[25] it relieves surgeons indefinitely of the responsibility of listening to any former patient.

If genital surgery is indeed "better now" and getting better all the time, that is actually a strong argument for allowing intersex children to be free of nonconsensual early surgery: when they are old enough, should they choose surgery, they will benefit from more than a decade of surgical advances. Moreover, were genital surgery performed only on patients old enough to make informed decisions, surgeons could benefit from patient feedback on the outcome as soon as healing is complete. Imagine how quickly surgery might improve under such circumstances!

WHEN IS A CLITORECTOMY
NOT A CLITORECTOMY?

Until the early 1970s, surgeons usually "feminized" intersex children via clitorectomy: they simply amputated the tip and part of the shaft of the clitoris. Today, surgeons use a more elaborate technique when "feminizing" intersex infants, and they bristle at any equation of their work with clitorectomy, which has come to be considered sexual mutilation and a violation of women's human rights. A wide variety of surgical techniques are used today—these are called clitoroplasty, or, more specifically, clitoral recession or clitoral reduction.

The distinction between "clitorectomy" and "clitoroplasty" is more political than technical. I have interviewed African women subjected to traditional clitorectomy and intersexed women subjected to medical clitorectomy. In both groups, some women are deprived of clitoral sensation and orgasm; some retain sensation in the clitoral stump; and some of these retain orgasmic response.

I have also interviewed women who have been subjected to a wide variety of clitoroplasty techniques: some retain some clitoral sensation; some retain orgasmic response; some are deprived of clitoral sensation and orgasm; and some are left with chronic pain. I see no trend for clitoroplasty to be less sexually mutilating than clitorectomy. If two women have been subjected to clitoral surgery and their sexual function damaged, ought the one whose surgery was labeled "clitoroplasty" feel less mutilated than the one whose surgery was labeled "clitorectomy"? African mothers, no less than American surgeons, act from a desire to care for their daughters. American surgeons, no less than African mothers, are misguided when they direct a knife at a child's clitoris.

The suffix "-ectomy" means to cut something out; it does not demand that an organ be totally removed. Nor does clitorectomy remove the entire clitoris: typically the crura (legs) and part of the shaft are left in place. Clitoroplasty often removes *more* clitoral tissue than does clitorectomy, and entails more extensive genital dissection and scarring.[26] Clitoroplasty attempts to preserve the tip, or glans, of the clitoris, on the theory that sexual function can thus be retained. But it aggressively removes the clitoral shaft—the very tissue that retains sensation and orgasmic function in some clitorectomized women. Researchers in human sexuality have long known that women masturbate by stimulating the clitoral shaft, not the glans.[27]

Further, genital stimulation usually consists primarily of friction, and extensive, deep scarring consequent to clitoroplasty or any genital surgery can render genital stimulation more uncomfortable or painful than pleasurable or erotic. The claim that such extensive cutting, removal, and relocation of any tissue could be done without altering or compromising sensation is simply untenable. Indeed, it is well known that surgeries using similar microsurgical techniques for reconstruction after trauma in adults (for example, facial reconstruction, or transfer of a toe to replace an amputated finger) result in sensation that is typically greatly reduced, altered in character, or even painful.

THE HYPOSPADIAS
SURGERY TREADMILL

As with clitoral surgery, surgeons insist that techniques for surgical correction of hypospadias (in which the "pee hole" opens not at the tip, but somewhere along the underside or at the base of the penis) have so improved that they need not listen to unhappy former patients. But the following sample of my discussions over the past year with parents of infants and toddlers paints a different picture:

My four-year-old son had his hypospadias surgery when he was one year old. Since then, he has had four additional operations, mainly as a result of the hole closing up due to scar tissue. One time, the original hole opened up and had to be corrected. Another time, the urethra ballooned near the hole and had to be corrected, and most recently, he was experiencing pain during urination because the hole was closing up due to the scar tissue. His urine stream is so messy that he cannot stand to pee.[28]

My 14-month-old recently underwent hypospadias repair. It failed; he now has two openings; the old one did not close. I wish I had [spoken to a support group] before consenting to the surgery. I feel terrible; now he has to undergo another surgery at two years old. Will he have diminished sexual feeling?[29]

My son had a hypospadias repair at age one; the first repair was botched. The doctor actually made the hypospadias hole larger than it was by cutting a slit between a dummy hole and the head down to the hypospadias hole, which was under the head. He also caused cosmetic damage to the shaft [pulled the skin tighter around the penis]. My son has had to have two other surgeries to cosmetically fix what the first doctor did, and has had recurrent urinary tract infections, one of which resulted in a week-long hospitalization and IV antibiotics. He has to squeeze urine out of a diverticulum every time he pees, and still gets urinary tract infections. I [want his doctor to] understand the pain and suffering my son has been through due to his actions.[30]

My five-year-old son has undergone two hypospadias surgeries to date. He frequently says things like I hate my dong [penis], I wish I was born a girl, et cetera. Can your recommend a therapist who specializes in gender dysphoria related to surgical trauma?[31]

My son had a hypospadias repair when he was eight months old. From the time I delivered him the doctor told me he would need to have surgery to correct this problem. He will be seven next week and the scarring is awful. I think he would have been better off not having the surgery. When I go back to the urologist he tells me it looks fine. My son realizes that it doesn't look right and he comments to that effect. What information or advice can you give me? I am at the end of my wits about this.[32]

Obviously, the claim that hypospadias surgeries today are highly successful is simply not true. If surgeons continue to ignore ethical and empirical challenges, I fear only lawsuits by anguished parents will slow the rush to surgery.

POSTCARDS FROM THE PARADIGM SHIFT

A number of clinicians have listened to the voices of intersex adults and are not only changing their practice, but working to re-educate their colleagues. One (who is not yet comfortable being identified) told me that after she had addressed a group of pediatric endocrinologists, one approached her to say, "I never thought we had any idea what the [expletive] we were doing with these kids, and now I know I was right." On another occasion, after she had shown the video *Hermaphrodites Speak!*[33] at a staff meeting, a nurse approached her to relate how saddened and moved she was. She had always wondered in private, she said, about "what we were doing to those children," but had kept her opinion to herself because "the doctors must have known what they were doing."[34]

One clinician told me that his colleague had presented a small follow up that indicated poor results in teenage girls subjected to early clitoroplasty. "I expected them to be embarrassed. Imagine my surprise," he wrote, when the audience at the pediatric endocrinology conference "turned on [his colleague] like vicious dogs."[35]

There are signs that even holdouts for the traditional model realize that it is indefensible. One prominent surgeon with many publications to his name agreed to be interviewed about his work on intersex children only under condition of anonymity, and with details changed to further protect his identity.[36] Alice Dreger has told me that she was unable to recruit anyone to defend the ethics of the traditional model for this book.

Two important books that investigate the medicalization of intersexuality and incorporate extensive coverage of the experiences of former patients have been published this past year.[37] The silence with which these past books have been greeted by the community of clinicians is deafening. When Dreger's book led to an editorial in the *New York Times* questioning the ethic of early genital surgeries,[38] a leader in pediatric endocrinology privately advised his colleagues that Dreger's goal was personal notoriety and that her work should be ignored.

CONCLUSION

Surgery does not produce "normal" looking genitals[39]—a fact immediately obvious to anyone who glances at the "after" photos claimed as successes in surgery journals or surgical training tapes (see figure 15-1).[40] Rather, what surgery does is to convey the clear message that "abnormal" genitals (including surgically reconstructed ones) are unacceptable. Surgery inflicts emotional harm by legitimating the idea that the child is not lovable unless "fixed" with medically unnecessary plastic surgery carrying significant risks. For example, Martha Coventry told the *New York Times,* "I'd be considered one of the success stories. I still have clitoral sensation, and I'm orgasmic." Nonetheless, she said, "it's taken me my whole life to come to terms with my body and not to feel such terrible shame."[41]

Finally, as ethicists have noted repeatedly, the argument that "surgery is better now" ignores the lack of informed consent and patients' autonomy inherent in the old model. The argument "Surgery is better now," combined with an insistence on operating during infancy, gives surgeons a perpetual license to ignore patients' needs and voices. When we stop thinking of our children born with atypical genitals as monsters, we will no longer risk their adult sexualities with nonconsensual, medically unnecessary genital surgeries.

ACKNOWLEDGMENT

This chapter first appeared in *The Journal of Clinical Ethics* 9, no. 4 (Winter 1998); © 1998 by *The Journal of Clinical Ethics*; used with permission.

NOTES

1. S. Kessler, *Lessons from the Intersexed* (Piscataway, N.J.: Rutgers University Press, 1998); A.D. Dreger, " 'Ambiguous Sex'—or Ambivalent Medicine? Ethical Issues in the Medical Treatment of Intersexuality," *Hastings Center Report* 28, no. 3 (1998): 24-35; R.A. Crouch, "Betwixt and Between: Reflections on Intersexuality," chapter 3 of this volume; K. Kipnis and M. Diamond, "Pediatric Ethics and the Surgical Assignment of Sex," chapter 17 of this volume.

2. R.A. Crouch, "Betwixt and Between," see note 1 above; S.E. Preves, "For the Sake of the Children: Destigmatizing Intersexuality," chapter 4 of this volume.

3. C. Chase, ed., "Special Issue on Intersexuality," *Chrysalis: The Journal of Transgressive Gender Identities* 2, no. 5 (Fall 1997/Winter 1998); C. Chase, *Her-*

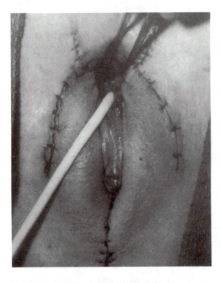

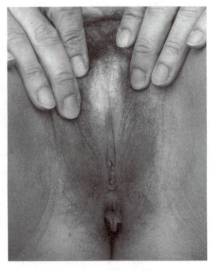

(A) "Appearance immediately after surgery, showing recession clitoroplasty and vaginal reconstruction. Note reconstruction of introitus using labioscrotal folds."

(B) "Clitorectomy" performed during childhood for "clitoral hypertrophy."

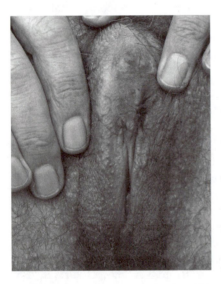

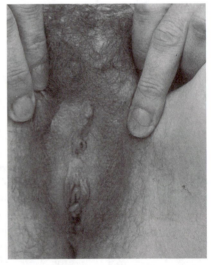

(C) "Clitoral recession" performed during childhood for "clitoral hypertrophy."

(D) "Clitoral recession" performed during childhood for "clitoral hypertrophy."

Figure 15-1.

Figure 15-1.

Surgeons' standards of normal appearance or cosmetic success are subjective judg-ments, and may differ from the judgments of laypeople, including their patients. Photo-graph (A) at left was presented by surgeons as a successful outcome. Reprinted from K. Newman, J. Randolph, and K. Anderson, "The Surgical Management of Infants and Chil-dren with Ambiguous Genitalia: Lessons Learned from 25 Years," *Annals of Surgery* 215, no. 6 (1992): 644-53, at 647, fig. 6, © 1992 by Lippincott Williams & Wilkins, used with permission.

Further, the appearance immediately after surgery may not reflect the appearance even a decade later. Pediatric urologist David Thomas noted, in a presentation to the American Academy of Pediatrics, that he has seen teenaged girls whose surgically recon-structed clitorises were quite visibly different from the original cosmetic result, with-ered, and obviously nonfunctional. D. Thomas, "Is Early Vaginal Reconstruction Wrong for Some Intersex Girls?" *Urology Times* (published by International Medical News), 10-12 February 1997.

Some intersexed adults have provided close-up photos of their genitals for the ex-plicit purpose of demonstrating how poor the surgical results are: photographs (B), (C), and (D); © 1998 by ISNA, used with permission.

---

maphrodites Speak! Intersex Society of North America (ISNA), 26 minutes, 1997, videocassette. Copies may be obtained from ISNA, PO Box 31791, San Fran-cisco, Calif. 94131; website <www.isna.org>.

4. M. Diamond and H.K. Sigmundson, "Management of Intersexuality: Guidelines for Dealing with Persons with Ambiguous Genitalia," *Archives of Pediatrics and Adolescent Medicine* 151 (1997): 1046-50. Text available from <www.afn.org/~sfcommed/apam.html>.

5. M. Hendricks, "Is It a Boy or a Girl?" *Johns Hopkins Magazine* (Novem-ber 1993): 10-16.

6. Dreger, " 'Ambiguous Sex'," see note 1 above.

7. Kipnis and Diamond, "Pediatric Ethics," see note 1 above; J.M. Schober, "Feminizing Genitoplasty for Intersex," in *Pediatric Surgery and Urology: Long-Term Outcomes*, ed. M.D. Stringer et al. (London: W.B. Saunders, 1998), 549-58.

8. J.K. Lattimer, "Relocation and Recession of the Enlarged Clitoris with Preservation of the Glans: An Alternative to Amputation," *Journal of Urology* 86, no. 1 (July 1961): 113-16.

9. Hendricks, "Is It a Boy," see note 5 above.

10. E. Barry, "United States of Ambiguity," *Boston Phoenix* (Styles section), 22 November 1996, 6-8.

11. G. Szasz and E. Durbach, "Becoming a Boy or a Girl," (Vancouver, B.C., Canada: British Columbia's Children's Hospital, 1995), 76.

12. N. Sagehashi, "Clitoroplasty for Clitoromegaly Due to Adrenogenital

Syndrome without Loss of Sensitivity," *Plastic and Reconstructive Surgery* 91, no. 5 (1993): 950-56.

13. M.T. Edgerton, "Discussion: Clitoroplasty for Clitoromegaly Due to Adrenogenital Syndrome without Loss of Sensitivity (by Nobuyuki Sagehashi)," *Plastic and Reconstructive Surgery* 91, no. 5 (1993): 956.

14. Sagehashi, "Clitoroplasty," see note 12 above; Edgerton, "Discussion: Clitoroplasty," see note 13 above.

15. Personal communication with the author by M. Edgerton, 1994.

16. Crouch, "Betwixt and Between," see note 1 above.

17. J.A. Talcott et al., "Patient-Reported Impotence and Incontinence after Nerve-Sparing Radical Prostatectomy," *Journal of the National Cancer Institute* 89, no. 15 (1997): 1117-23.

18. C. Chase, "Re: Measurement of Evoked Potentials during Feminizing Genitoplasty: Techniques and Applications" (letter), *Journal of Urology* 156, no. 3 (1996): 1139-40.

19. A.C. Kinsey et al., *Sexual Behavior in the Human Female* (Philadelphia: W.B. Saunders, 1953).

20. Personal communication with the author by J. Randolph, 1993.

21. Personal communication with the author by a surgeon who asked to remain anonymous, 1998.

22. Personal communication with the author by a pediatric endocrinologist who asked to remain anonymous.

23. S.A. Groveman, "The Hannukah Bush," chapter 2 of this volume.

24. Kipnis and Diamond, "Pediatric Ethics," see note 1 above.

25. Crouch, "Betwixt and Between," see note 1 above.

26. J.E. Oesterling, J.P. Gearhart, and R.D. Jeffs, "A Unified Approach to Early Reconstructive Surgery of the Child with Ambiguous Genitalia," *Journal of Urology* 138 (1987): 1079-84.

27. Kinsey et al., *Sexual Behavior in the Human Female*, see note 19 above.

28. Personal communication with the author by a mother who asked to remain anonymous, 21 June 1998.

29. Personal communication with the author by a parent who asked to remain anonymous, 11 January 1998.

30. Personal communication with the author by a parent who asked to remain anonymous, 4 September 1997.

31. Personal communication with the author by a parent who asked to remain anonymous, 15 August 1997.

32. Personal communication with the author by a parent who asked to remain anonymous, 24 June 1997.

33. See note 3 above.

34. Personal communication with the author by an endocirinologist who asked to remain anonymous.

35. Personal communication with the author by Nicholas Johnson.

36. E.H.-J. Lee, "Producing Sex: An Interdisciplinary Perspective on Sex Assignment Decisions for Intersexuals" (Senior thesis, Brown University, 1994).

37. Kessler, *Lessons from the Intersexed,* see note 1 above; A.D. Dreger, *Hermaphrodites and the Medical Invention of Sex* (Cambridge, Mass.: Harvard University Press, 1998).

38. A. Dreger, "When Medicine Goes Too Far in the Pursuit of Normality," *New York Times* (Science Times), 28 July 1998.

39. C. Migeon, "Outcomes in Androgen Insensitivity Syndrome" (Data presented at the Lawson Wilkins Pediatric Endocrinology Society Annual Meeting, San Francisco, 30 April 1999).

40. See, for example, R. Hurwitz, H. Applebaum, and S. Muenchow, *Surgical Reconstruction of Ambiguous Genitalia in Female Children,* ACS/USSC Educational Library, no. ACS-1613, 21 minutes, 1990 videocassette. Copies may be obtained from Cine-Med, 127 Main St. North, P.O. Box 745, Woodbury, Conn. 06798; telephone (800) 633-0004.

41. N. Angier, "New Debate Over Surgery on Genitals," *New York Times,* 13 May 1997, B7.

16

A Surgeon's Response to the Intersex Controversy

Justine Marut Schober

Alice Domurat Dreger asked several prominent surgeons who treat intersexed patients to write for this volume. Dr. Schober was the only surgeon willing to do so. Her article addresses five key questions articulated by Dr. Dreger.

QUESTION 1

Do you think people should have the right to make decisions about cosmetic genital surgeries that risk their sexual pleasure, function, and fertility?

Not only do they have the right, they are the *only* persons who have the authority to make such a personal decision. Increasing awareness of dissatisfaction after gender assignment surgery, particularly feminizing surgery, has made surgeons very cautious. Loss of sexual sensation, orgasmic potential, and sexual function are particularly disturbing, considering that these problems may result from the surgery itself.

QUESTION 2

What are the specific goals of intersex treatment and how do current treatment methods address these goals?

Our goal in intersex treatment has never changed: to facilitate a patient's positive psychosocial and psychosexual adjustment throughout life. As surgeons, we have addressed the aesthetic appearance and functionality of the external genitalia with the belief that the physical changes we impose would help increase psychosocial and psychosexual comfort. Medical and surgical therapies have changed in both timing and refinement. Physical treatment has been offered in two categories: surgery and/ or hormonal intervention. The immediate aesthetic results seem to continually improve. However, the long-term efficacy of the structural results of various surgeries and their impact on the individual's psychological, social, and physical adjustment remain unknown.

Surgery to change the appearance of the genitalia dependably achieves masculinizing or feminizing appearance, with low immediate risks and good aesthetic outcomes. Currently, we can correct severe hypospadias and provide a very good masculinized appearance, with less reoperation. Surgical techniques may make these individuals who have corresponding masculine gender recognition more comfortable with their body image. Because we do not remove tissue, sexual sensation has probably not been affected.

In feminizing surgery, two longer-term outcomes other than aesthetics are involved in sexual functioning: creating a long-lasting vagina to allow penetration for intercourse and preserving sensation for orgasmic response. Success of vaginoplasty varies with type. When foreign tissues are used, vaginal cancer may occur at younger ages, but the incidence of this is rare.[1] Preservation of sensation and function is currently being investigated. Patient commentary suggests that sexual sensitivity may be altered.[2]

In 1995, Gearhart reported preserved nerve latency in patients two to 23 months of age who had undergone clitoroplasty with preservation of the neuro-vascular bundle. However, this does not prove preservation of sexual sensation or guarantee normal adult sexual function.[3] Chase refutes nerve conduction studies, citing an adult patient with normal nerve conduction and no sexual sensitivity.[4]

Long-term studies have not yet addressed the intersexual person's body image, socialization, or relationship to parents. Many surgeons believe that parents would have a difficult, if not impossible, time rearing a child who was assigned female but appeared virilized, or vice versa. Societal attitudes would also presumably make adjustment difficult for such a child, subjecting him/her to teasing and ostracism. These and other factors are often used to justify early gender-determining surgery. Many surgeons believe that the surgery is easier and more successful if performed very early. Early surgery addresses parental comfort and a societal view of what constitutes either a male or female genital appearance. Whether genital appearance significantly impacts a firm gender conviction remains undetermined. Masculinizing or feminizing surgery may make an individual more comfortable in situations where the genitalia are exposed (that is, sexually interactive situations or changing clothes in another's presence).

Little factual evidence or long-term outcome studies exist to guide choices. This represents one of the biggest problems regarding early surgery for intersexuals. Mounting evidence suggests patients' dissatisfaction with surgery on the genitalia, citing problems such as gender dysphoria (genitals do not reflect the patient's development of gender identity) and lack of sexual sensation after feminizing surgeries. This has occurred with both old-fashioned clitorectomy and the newer forms of reduction clitoroplasty. Delaying a surgical choice to allow patients' input increases the probability of surgery matching gender identity and gives the patient a choice of what risks are acceptable if he/she wishes aesthetic or functional changes.

Surgeons have always given parents of minors the right to accept or refuse medical advice on behalf of their children. Herein lies the ethical problem. In these cases, functional outcomes are not apparent until many years after the actual surgery. The outcomes are very personal, not something that can be chosen for another person. We cannot predict with confidence what a child's gender preference will be. How could anyone make a decision for another when the decision trades appearance at the risk of lessened or absent sexual sensation? For the best long-term outcomes, we need to consider that surgical treatment methods do not "cure" intersexuality, and that a procedure such as vaginoplasty should address a consenting and requesting patient's needs and desires, not parental and societal comfort.

QUESTION 3

Is it true that doctors sometimes withhold information from intersexuals and their parents? Do you ever think it ethical to withhold information?

To help parents arrive at a rational decision, most doctors try to provide information they believe parents could best comprehend. Obviously, the amount and quality of information provided or withheld varies greatly. Though withholding information may be well intended, this is not always best in the long run.

Parents and patients have become more aware, more educated, and proactive in recent years. This has forced doctors to realize that the information that is discussed needs to be truthful and complete. Years ago, a doctor would do what he thought best for patient and parents without involving them in decision making. In the past, this was considered highly appropriate and ethical, but it is no longer true.

Medical diagnoses and records are readily available to both patient and parent, making withholding information potentially harmful, illegal, and unethical. We desire the easiest psychological adjustment for a patient. Though deception might allow an easier adjustment in some cases, the parent and patient have a right to know, as well as the right to make educated, prospective choices. The doctor has the responsibility to provide complete information and to take time with parents to ensure optimal understanding of the information. This includes discussions regarding short- and long-term outcomes. Providing access to support groups facilitates adjustment to intersexuality. The support group can provide unique insight and a more human perspective on the challenges related to this condition.

When dealing with intersexuality, doctors may also encounter a problem with parents who request that information be withheld from a child. I truly believe that withholding information breaks a trust and will eventually create bigger problems when and if the condition comes to light. I believe doctors should caution parents against this, citing difficulty in relationships once an affected individual realizes he/she has been deceived. If deceived, a patient may feel distrustful of the parents and the entire medical establishment.

I recently reviewed a paper about clinical management of androgen insensitivity syndrome (AIS), written by a person with AIS. The author suggested that she believed the most critical recommendation was that the physician encourage the parents to tell the child the truth. Otherwise, the child may experience deep feelings of shame resulting from an aura of secrecy that accompanies such deception. If the patient senses that both parents and doctors accept and are comfortable with the diagnosis, the long-term prospects for emotional healing and stability are greatly increased. Withholding information encourages secrecy and may ultimately lead to confusion, frustration, and isolation more damaging than the diagnosis.[5]

QUESTION 4

Do you feel there is adequate evidence to support the treatment protocols to which many surgeons subscribe (for example, surgically altering, in infancy or childhood, XY micropenis children's genitals to more closely approximate a feminine anatomy)? If so, what is the evidence?

In many cases, very little evidence currently exists to either support or refute surgery. However, recommendations are becoming less controversial for certain diagnostic groups. For example, when a child is diagnosed with micropenis and normal male chromosomes, more evidence is available to support rearing this child as male, despite small genital size. Long-term studies report that these boys can have normal male gender recognition and normal sensation, erectile capacity, orgasm, and fertility.[6]

Good evidence also exists to support surgical therapy in cases of severe XY penoscrotal hypospadias [a condition in which the urethra opens on the underside of the penis—*ED.*]. In one- or two-stage repairs performed between the ages of six and 15 months, the surgical outcomes are excellent. Psychosexual and psychosocial development of children, adolescents, and adults after hypospadias surgery has been found to be normal in general.[7]

Evidence is increasing to support male gender rearing in boys with cloacal exstrophy. These boys have normal XY chromosomes, but may lack a penis; however, testes are usually present. Studies by Reiner suggest that they will likely exhibit more male-type behaviors, with sexual orientation toward females. Even if the child is reared female, with XY chromosomes and androgen from normal testes, the brain may be masculinized. Surgical construction of a phallus is possible, with relatively good aesthetic results. Unfortunately, spontaneous erection is not yet possible and orgasmic potential is questionable, as it would be regardless of sex of rearing.[8]

In complete forms of androgen insensitivity syndrome, where feminized external genitalia exist with normal male (XY) chromosomes, affected children seem only to identify as females. Patients lack a uterus, ovaries, and a normal vagina. Testes are present, but usually undescended. I feel long-term outcomes support female rearing, but controversy exists on timing of orchidectomy [surgical excision of the testes—*ED.*]. Consideration must be given to testicular tumor potential, though this is rare before puberty.[9] Delaying orchidectomy will allow spontaneous female development at puberty via conversion of endogenous testosterone to estradiol, and the patient's involvement in decision making. An alternative would be early orchidectomy with administration of estrogen; however, this may lead to early osteoporosis.

Controversy also continues regarding timing of vaginoplasty. Little evidence exists to guide timing. I would once again defer to the patient's choice for both timing and type of vaginoplasty.

The diagnosis of 46XX congenital adrenal hyperplasia (CAH) can generally be quickly established by demonstrating elevated plasma 17-hydroxyprogesterone. Patients have a female karyotype with normal female internal genitalia (uterus and ovaries present). These children are traditionally raised as girls, though they may have significantly masculinized brain development. They also have varying degrees of genital masculinization. Reduction of an enlarged clitoris and, in some cases, vaginoplasty has been the traditional response, but potential damage to sensation and reduced orgasmic potential is again tendered. In those girls with complete virilization, sexual orientation is unpredictable. Currently, we think some may adjust better as males.[10]

Curiously, the greatest number of published reports regarding long-term outcomes are available for this diagnosis. The surgical and clinical complications of the patients with 46XX CAH may account for lower quality of life scores. CAH patients were more often single (66 percent), with fewer children than controls. Homosexual preference was not increased, suggesting either avoidance of close personal relationships[11] or possible problems with data collection.

Beyond these diagnoses, very little long-term evidence exists regarding treatment of infants and children with mixed gonadal dysgenesis, male pseudo-hermaphroditism, or true hermaphroditism.

Reiner suggests these individuals may demonstrate more male-type behaviors that may be accentuated with testosterone in the first few months of life. Pubescent androgen levels will most likely also accentuate male behavior. Again, removal of gonadal/testicular tissue in intersex patients with a Y chromosome is recommended because of the strong association of the genesis of tumor in dysgenetic gonads. Timing in these cases is earlier than in AIS because of higher percentages of tumor formation at earlier ages.[12]

QUESTION 5

Do you think intersexuals and their parents should be given information about support groups by clinicians?
I think support groups serve a vital, important purpose. They represent the only source that can provide authoritative counsel to parents and patients of exactly how it feels to be in such a situation: their reaction to social and medical situations or to surgery versus conservative management. I think it is comforting for both family and patient to identify with others similarly affected and to see that such a child can mature

into a successful, functioning adult. This is something that a parent desperately needs when confronted with a situation whose outcome she or he cannot imagine. Parents' immediate, overwhelming concern is what their child will grow up to look and act like. Being able to talk to adults with an intersexual condition and parents of intersexual children may be more reassuring than any words of encouragement a physician can offer. Also, seeing that an adult is able to thrive, despite knowledge of the condition, will make parents more secure as they raise their children. For patients themselves, one of the most difficult aspects of intersexuality may be feeling different and alone in the world. Discussion with patients in several support groups showed the commonality of these feelings. They found coping much easier if they had opportunities to meet other intersexuals.

ACKNOWLEDGMENT

This chapter first appeared in *The Journal of Clinical Ethics* 9, no. 4 (Winter 1998); © 1998 by *The Journal of Clinical Ethics*; used with permission.

NOTES

1. R.N. Ritchie, "Primary Carcinoma of the Vagina Following a Baldwin Reconstruction Operation for Congenital Absence of the Vagina," *American Journal of Obstetrics and Gynecology* 18 (1929): 794; P. Lavand-Homme, "Late Carcinoma of the Artificial Vagina Formed from the Rectum," *Bruxelles Medical* 19 (1938): 14; E. Adryjowicz et al., "Adenocarcinoma in a Cecal Neovagina—Complication of Irradiation: Report of a Case and Review of Literature," *Gynecologic Oncology* 21, no. 2 (June 1985): 235-39; M. Ursic-Vrscaj et al., "Adenocarcinoma in a Sigmoid Neovagina 22 Years after Wertheim-Meigs Operation. Case Report," *European Journal of Gynaecological Oncology* 15, no. 1 (1994): 24-28; G.W. Jackson, "Primary Carcinoma of an Artificial Vagina," *Obstetrics and Gynecology* 14, no. 4 (October 1959): 534-36.

2. C. Chase, "Letter of Response," *Journal of Urology* 156, no. 3 (1996): 1139-40.

3. J.P. Gearhart, A. Burnett, and J.H. Owen, "Measurement of Pudendal Evoked Potentials During Feminizing Genitoplasty: Technique and Applications," *Journal of Urology* 153 (February 1995): 486-87.

4. Chase, "Letter of Response," see note 2 above.

5. Personal communication: Sherri A. Groveman and J.D. Groveman, "Clinical Management of Complete Androgen Insensitivity Syndrome: The Patient's Perspective."

6. J.M. Reilly and C.R.J. Woodhouse, "Small Penis and the Male Sexual

Role," *Journal of Urology* 142 (August 1989): 569-71.

7. M.A. Mureau et al., "Psychologic Functioning of Children, Adolescents, and Adults Following Hypospadias Surgery: a Comparative Study," *Journal of Pediatric Psychology* 22, no. 3 (June 1997): 371-87.

8. W.G. Reiner, "Sex Assignment in the Neonate with Intersex or Inadequate Genitalia," *Archives of Pediatrics and Adolescent Medicine* 151, no. 10 (October 1997): 1044-45.

9. M. Manuel, K.P. Katayoma, and H.W. Jones, "The Age of Occurrence of Gonadal Tumors in Intersex Patients with a Y Chromosome," *American Journal of Obstetrics and Gynecology* 124, no. 3 (February 1976): 293-300.

10. Reiner, "Sex Assignment," see note 8 above.

11. U. Kuhnle, M. Bullinger, and H.P. Schwarz, "The Quality of Life in Adult Female Patients with Congenital Adrenal Hyperplasia: A Comprehensive Study of the Impact of Genital Malformations and Chronic Disease on Female Patients' Life," *European Journal of Pediatrics* 154 (1995): 708-16.

12. Manuel et al., "The Age of Occurrence," see note 9 above.

PART 4

What to Do Now

Introduction to Part 4

The essays of this section explicitly address the question, "Where do we go from here?"—a question that, of course, has been at least implicitly addressed by virtually all of the preceding chapters. (Alice Domurat Dreger's essay summarizes the elements that most of the authors in this volume think need to be included in the new intersex management paradigm; see chapter 1).

In the first chapter of this section, ethicist Kenneth Kipnis and sexologist Milton Diamond make three strong recommendations: first, that there be a general moratorium on medically unnecessary surgeries when they are done without the consent of the intersexed patient him/herself; second, that this moratorium not be lifted unless in-depth follow-up studies show that the surgeries have been efficacious from the patients' point of view; third, that efforts be made to undo the effects of clinicians' lying to or withholding the truth from intersexed patients.

These recommendation are supplemented by "A Mother's 10 Commandments to Medical Professionals: Treating Intersex in the Newborn," offered by Helena Harmon-Smith, a mother of an intersexed child and the founder of a support group for parents of intersexuals. An autobiographical essay by an intersexed adult, Heidi Walcutt, follows Harmon-Smith's piece. Walcutt and Harmon-Smith each draw on their own experiences to suggest immediate steps that clinicians can take to avoid traumatizing intersexed children and their families.

In a darkly humorous essay entitled "Take Charge! A Guide to Home Autocatheterization," Sven Nicholson—a man confined to life-long catheterization because of surgeries designed to "normalize" the appearance of his penis—documents how he has learned to self-medicate and so to wrestle himself free of the medical establishment. Nicholson suggests this kind of self-treatment for other intersexuals who are tired of the medical treadmill.

Finally, Edmund Howe closes the volume with several innovative suggestions for how clinicians could start treating the psychosocial problem of intersex as a psychosocial problem. He argues for the need to bring intersex practice into line with the underlying goal—a goal with which virtually everyone agrees—"For these children, as they grow up, to be happy."

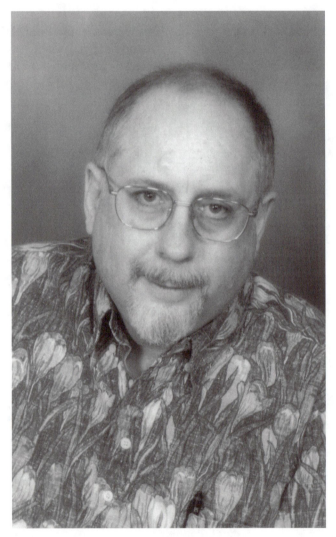

Kenneth Kipnis

17

Pediatric Ethics and the Surgical Assignment of Sex

Kenneth Kipnis and Milton Diamond

It has been standard pediatric practice to recommend surgery for infants with ambiguous genitalia or loss of the penis. The parents of these patients are told to raise them without ambiguity and, in consequence, many adults who have had these operations in infancy have never been candidly informed of their medical histories. This management approach, which can involve a reassignment of sex, has its basis in research done on hermaphrodites and a single set of nonhermaphroditic identical twins originally tracked more than two decades ago. The current article reviews this practice and its epistemic foundations. It is argued that there should be a moratorium on such surgery; that the medical profession should complete comprehensive look-back studies to assess the outcomes of past interventions; and that efforts should be made to undo the effects of past deception.

CASE REPORT

In 1983, one of the authors of this study (KK) received a call from a pediatric surgeon to do a clinical ethics consultation following the birth of a full-term baby boy with multiple congenital anomalies. While other deficits will be described below, the surgeon was immediately concerned about the child's abnormally small penis: technically, a micropenis. Apprehensive about the possibility of the child being shamed in the boys'

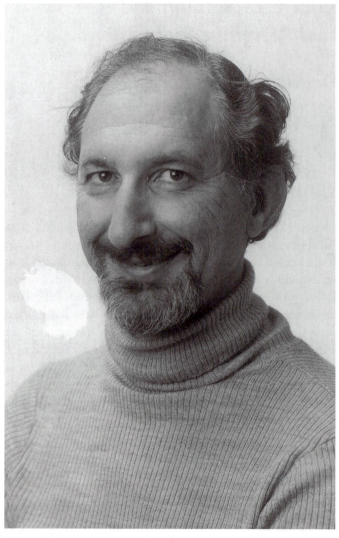

Milton Diamond

locker room—psychosocial distress as he matured—the pediatric surgeon was counseling immediate surgical reassignment as a girl. According to the surgeon's plan, the testes would be removed and the genitalia fashioned into a cosmetic vulva before the baby left the hospital. The parents would be instructed to raise the infant as an unambiguous girl. At about the age of 12, estrogens would be administered to stimulate the development of female secondary sex characteristics. Eventually doctors would create an artificial vagina. Although the resulting woman would be unable to bear children, the surgeon anticipated that prompt surgical attention would allow the infant to enjoy a better and more normal life as a female than would be possible for a male with a very small penis.

The boy's mother was livid with rage and bitterness. Having given birth only days earlier, her dreams of a perfect child had disintegrated into a nightmarish reality. Pronouns were failing her and she did not know what to say to relatives. Communication had broken down with the surgeon and she was unable to discuss reassignment with him much less consent to it. It fell to the ethics consultant to try to resolve the impasse by investigating the issues and making a recommendation. Research went in two directions: a survey of the literature on ambiguous genitalia and an inquiry into the medical condition of the infant. It was in the context of this case that the authors of the present article first began to work together: the philosopher-ethicist consulted with his colleague (MD) across the campus at the John A. Burns School of Medicine.

The literature review led immediately to the work of John Money, then a psychologist at the Gender Identity Clinic at the Johns Hopkins University. In a series of articles and a landmark 1972 book (*Man & Woman, Boy & Girl*),[1] Money and Anka Ehrardt described the case of a pair of identical male twins born in the 1960s. At the age of seven months, the boys were scheduled for circumcision because of phimosis (a narrowing of the opening of the foreskin). An electrocautery knife used on one of the boys severely burned his penis, destroying it. A psychiatrist at the time expressed what one supposes was the conventional wisdom about the boys probable future: "He will be unable to consummate marriage or have normal heterosexual relations; he will have to recognize that he is incomplete, physically defective, and that he must live apart."[2]

Crushed by the loss, the parents learned of Money's work at Johns Hopkins and the early sex-change operations that were being done there. Following consultation, Money recommended to the parents that the boy be surgically reassigned and raised as a girl. Accordingly, at the age of 17 months, surgeons removed his testes and reshaped his scrotum to approximate a vulva. John, as he later became known in the literature, had become Joan, to be raised as a normal girl without any suspicion of early trauma.

Money's earlier research had convinced him that hermaphroditic children who appeared physiologically similar to each other could none-theless develop into adults identifying and behaving either as men or as women.[3] Inferring from this work that all infants are sexually neutral at birth and malleable during a window period that remains open until about 18 to 24 months when gender becomes fixed, Money concluded that social imprinting and learning were the key factors in psychosexual development: an account that was consistent with research in language acquisition. Finally, echoing Freud,[4] Money surmised that the presence or absence of the penis was the critical anatomical factor. In a nutshell, the theory held that sexually neutral infants, both consciously and sub-consciously, notice the presence or absence of a penis, observe the social distinctions between males and females, and characteristically comport with local standards of gender. Thus, given an unambiguous upbringing, normal behavior would follow perceived anatomy. While earlier reports had described the reassignment of infants with ambiguous genitalia, the appearance of unambiguously male identical twins, one needing atten-tion, offered an unparalleled opportunity to confirm the theory of sexual neutrality at birth.

The twins were evaluated regularly at Hopkins and, in a series of celebrated publications,[5] Money described their psychosexual develop-ment to about the onset of puberty: the one surgically reassigned as a girl and the other identical twin, in effect, a control. Glowingly relating re-markable results, Money wrote in 1975: "No one . . . would . . . ever conjecture [that Joan was born a boy]. Her behavior is so normally that of an active little girl, and so clearly different by contrast from the boy-ish ways of her twin brother, that it offers nothing to stimulate one's conjectures."[6] Reported in professional publications and the national media,[7] Money's writings dramatically confirmed the plasticity of gen-der: an infant, born as an unambiguous male, had been surgically reas-signed as female and successfully reared as a normal girl.

Drawing on Money's research and his theory of psychosexual devel-opment, pediatricians caring for infants with ambiguous genitalia inferred that genetic makeup and prenatal endocrinology could largely be ignored in the clinical assignment of sex. They reasoned that the penis had to be plainly absent or present from infancy on, and that these children had to be raised as girls or boys with no hint of abnormality. Accordingly, pediatric surgeons would strive to benefit these patients by "normalizing" ambiguous genitalia: reducing enlarged clitorides (eliminating visible penis-like structures in babies assigned as females) and, because of the technical difficulty of creating functional and cosmetically believable male genitals, refashioning anomalous male genitalia as female.

Well before the 1983 birth of the boy with micropenis, Money's published work had emerged as the epistemic foundation for the new pediatric standard of practice. Thus it was clear why the surgeon wanted to reassign the baby boy as a girl. Pediatric textbooks, then and now, characteristically recommend surgery when the size of the stretched penis is less than about 2.0 centimeters[8] or when the size of the clitoris is greater than about 1 centimeter.[9] If surgical disambiguation could succeed with an infant born unambiguously male, it would—it was thought—surely benefit other babies with ambiguous genitalia. These medical interventions, done with parental consent, as soon after birth as possible, were taken as beneficial, like the pediatric correction of cleft palate. The hermaphrodite and twin studies, it was thought, provided evidence that surgery benefited children with ambiguous genitalia and that, eventually, as one would suppose for infants with cleft palate, they too would have reason to thank their parents and doctors for medical ministrations received as infants.

In this case, while the literature supported the surgeon's 1983 recommendation, doubts arose following inquiry into other aspects of the boy's medical condition. There were other congenital anomalies. A second physician called attention to the boy's undeveloped eyes; the baby was blind. There was evidence of deafness and a probability of other central nervous system deficits, the nature and extent of which had not yet been determined. Accordingly, the child was unlikely to experience locker-room derision and might even go through life without being conscious of gender. The ethics consultant concluded that surgery could not be expected to benefit this particular patient and recommended that reassignment be delayed indefinitely. The surgeon and the parents concurred and the procedure was not done.

While more can be said about this case, here we want to observe both the narrowness of the clinical vision—the focus of attention initially did not extend above the pubis—and the mechanical application of a standard of practice calling for surgical reassignment on the basis of micropenis. We will revisit these themes below.

THE FURTHER HISTORY OF JOHN/JOAN

Notwithstanding that Money and Ehrardt's twin study had only a single experimental subject and a single control, such publications were nonetheless decisive in establishing what quickly became the standard of practice in pediatrics. As recently as April of 1996, the American Academy of Pediatrics (AAP) issued recommendations governing the "Timing of Elective Surgery on the Genitalia of Male Children . . . ":

Research on children with ambiguous genitalia has shown that sexual identity is a function of social learning through differential responses of multiple individuals in the environment. For example, children whose genetic sexes are not clearly reflected in external genitalia (i.e., hermaphroditism) can be raised successfully as members of either sex if the process begins before the age of 2 years. Therefore, a person's sexual body image is largely a function of socialization.[10]

The three works cited by the AAP in support of these findings list John Money as the lead author. No corroborating research is referenced. In fact, Money's theory and recommendations had been vigorously challenged in medical and scientific literature.[11] Suzanne Kessler has written: "Almost all of the published literature on intersexed infant case management has been written or co-written by one researcher, John Money. . . . Even though psychologists fiercely argue issues of gender identity and gender role development, doctors who treat intersexed infants seem untouched by those debates. . . . Why Money has been so single-handedly successful in promoting his ideas about gender is a question worthy of a separate substantial analysis."[12]

It is worthwhile to note that as early as 1966, medicine was coming to terms with transsexuals, individuals whose sexual self-identification is in opposition to their genital configuration and rearing.[13] Despite appropriate anatomy and socialization, the existence of these adults should have stimulated the AAP to question its acceptance that "sexual identity is a function of social learning."

It is conservatively estimated that one in 2,000 newborns are found to have ambiguous external genitalia,[14] that 100 to 200 pediatric surgical sex reassignments are performed in the United States annually, and that, globally, thousands of these procedures have been done since the initial publication of the twins case.[15] It is notable that, notwithstanding more than three decades of clinical experience with the surgical reassignment of infants, there have been no systematic, large-scale studies done to assess the outcome of these procedures. (Some small-scale reviews have been done by Kessler,[16] Schober,[17] and others noted below.) It is also notable that Money's narrative of the twins case ends before his subjects reach adolescence. In his last update, in 1978, Money writes: "Now prepubertal in age, the girl has . . . a feminine gender identity and role distinctly different from that of her brother. . . . The final and conclusive evidence awaits the appearance of romantic interest and erotic imagery."[18] This evidence never appears, and John/Joan, like many of these patients, is "lost to follow-up."

While several recent developments have called into question the venerable basis for the standard of pediatric practice, perhaps the most dramatic has been the reopening of the John/Joan case. In 1994, one of the authors of this study (MD) located and interviewed the former research subject. A richer and more comprehensive picture has emerged of the childhood that loomed so prominently in the literature of the 1970s.[19]

The child never was and never became a normal girl. Now in his thirties, having married a woman with three children, John lives as a man. He, his mother, and his brother now recall that Joan regularly rejected girls' toys, clothes, and activities. His mother says that, despite an attractive female appearance, Joan's movements and speech "gave him away and the awkwardness and incongruities became apparent."[20] John's twin brother has said: "When I say there was nothing feminine about Joan, I mean there was *nothing* feminine. She talked about guy things, didn't give a crap about cleaning house, getting married, wearing makeup" [emphasis in original]. At the age of six or seven, Joan told her brother she wanted to be a garbage man: "Easy job, good pay."[21] Despite the absence of a penis, Joan often stood to urinate. Other girls at school eventually barred her from their bathroom, threatening to kill her if she came in. Eventually she would use a back alley for urination.[22] Contrary to Money's earlier reports, Joan's behavior during childhood failed to be "so normally that of an active little girl."

Despite rearing as a girl, Joan dreamed of a future as a he-man type with a mustache and sports car. Although placed on estrogens at the age of 12, she often discarded the drugs, disliking how they made her feel. She was disturbed by her developing breasts. At one point she told her endocrinologist that she had suspected she was a boy since the second grade. She adamantly refused the surgery that would give her a vagina and complained to her psychiatrist how she dreaded the trips to Johns Hopkins where people looked at her and showed her pictures of nude bodies. At the conclusion of her final visit in 1978, Joan told her mother she would kill herself if she had to go again. By 1980 Joan's relationship with her clinicians at Hopkins had reached an impasse. "Do you want to be a girl or not?" her endocrinologist had demanded. "No!" replied Joan emphatically. At the age of 14, without knowing the history, she decided to cease living as a girl: Joan became John.[23]

Following the transition, John's father, on the advice of a psychiatrist, revealed what had happened during infancy. Until that moment her parents and clinicians had tried to conceal all that was problematic about her gender, to give her the unambiguous rearing as a girl they were told to provide. Listening intently to his father tell the story of the botched circumcision and surgery, John experienced relief. A puzzling past began to make sense. At John's request, male hormones were subsequently administered, a mastectomy was performed, and surgeons eventually created a penis. John now takes satisfaction as a husband, father, and breadwinner.

In retrospect, it seems clear that the surgical refashioning of infants' genitalia must be assessed during the adulthoods of those patients, after the sexual organs take on their distinctive importance in intimate and procreative relationships. To judge success by genital appearance and psychosexual development prior to puberty is to fall victim to narrowed vision.[24] When viewed comprehensively, the life of John/Joan undercuts both the standard of practice and the theory that children observe the distinction between male and female and comport with local standards of gender. Though Joan learned all she was supposed to, her behavior nonetheless exhibited quintessential male elements, and she failed to identify as female. Feminine social imprinting did not occur. In the end, the medical intervention had added the insults of infertility, emotional trauma, and ego loss to the injury of an accidental penectomy. Castration now necessitates a continuing regimen of male hormone replacement.

OTHER DEVELOPMENTS

The outcome of the John/Joan case has been observed with comparable patients. In a recent and ongoing study, Reiner tracked six boys who had lost their penises in infancy and were being reared as girls. These children behaved more like boys than girls and, in two cases, not knowing they were XY, the children autonomously changed gender and assumed male roles.[25] Reiner has stated: "it would be wrong to say that these two children wished to be boys or felt they were boys in girls' bodies: they believed they were boys."[26]

Another significant development has been the emergence of the Intersex Society of North America (ISNA) and related advocacy and support groups. The ISNA membership includes adults who were surgically "normalized" as children, generally without being told, and other intersexuals who have not had surgery. Having attempted unsuccessfully to dialogue with medical organizations in the U.S., some intersexuals have taken to picketing hospitals and conferences.[27] Unlike those with surgically corrected cleft palates, intersex patients are condemning physicians for their surgeries and for withholding the truth about their medical condition and treatment. The John/Joan case, the Reiner study, the activist protests, and other cases reported in the literature[28] strongly suggest that pediatric reassignment may often be failing the "thank you test" for clinical beneficence,[29] and that these poor outcomes may not be isolated droplets of misfortune in a downpour of excellent results.

There is some research exploring what happens when infants do not receive surgery. One well-known outcome study has been done on adult males with micropenis who would have been reassigned in infancy as females under the present standard of practice. While six of these 12 postpubertal males admitted to having been teased about a small penis, all "felt male," were gynecophilic, and had erections and orgasms. Nine had sexual intercourse satisfactory to themselves and their partners; seven were married or cohabiting, and still others were sexually active. One had become a father.[30] Another study reported success in helping men with very small penises who presented at a clinic for counseling. All were sexually functional. They and their partners were able to come to terms with their differences.[31] Contrary to conventional wisdom, it is not inevitable that such a man must "recognize that he is incomplete, physically defective, and that he must live apart."

The locker-room argument—that an individual without a penis would be subject to ridicule by peers—has recently received attention. A preoperative female-to-male transsexual has related showering routines that allow one to manage without embarrassment.[32]

A review of the literature has failed to turn up a single article on the hazards, psychosocial or otherwise, of having a large clitoris.[33] Most individuals are not aware that a size standard exists and, indeed, in some cases the parents were unaware of the presence of their daughters' hypertrophied clitoris until clinicians pointed it out in the context of recommending surgery.[34] On the contrary, there are reports of such women and their sexual partners enjoying the configuration (personal cases of MD). For women who have had the surgery, some retain a capacity for

orgasm[35] while others complain about pain and insensitivity.[36] Research
has not shown that any of the reduction procedures in use reliably preserve full erotic sensitivity into adulthood.

Finally, Kessler has polled adult men and women on their attitudes
toward surgery in infancy.[37] Women were asked if they would want surgical correction had they been born with a clitoris 1.0 to 2.5 centimeters;
93 percent said they would not have wanted treatment unless the condition was life threatening and the surgery would not reduce pleasurable
sensitivity. Over half of the women would not have wanted the surgery
even if the condition were unattractive and made them feel uncomfortable; 12 percent of the women would not have wanted the surgery under
any circumstance. Men were likewise asked whether they would want
reassignment as a female had they been born with micropenis. Over half
would not have wanted the reassignment under any condition. Almost
all would have refused surgery if it reduced pleasurable sensitivity or
orgasmic capability. The responses of Kessler's subjects are consistent
with the reasonable view that the roles that procreative capacity and
sexual pleasure play in intimate adult relationships are far more important than the normality of genital appearance. Despite dissent,[38] the pediatric standard of practice makes precisely the opposite ranking.

SEX AND GENDER

The conceptual distinction between male and female persons (men/
women, boys/girls, ladies/gentlemen, etcetera) is standard cognitive equip-
ment in culture, deeply implicated in self-identification and social ideol-
ogy. Particularly in the West, it is taken for granted that humanity comes
in two mutually exclusive sexes, and that these are readily distinguishable at birth by the presence or absence of a penis, which, in turn, signals
a vast array of other permanent physiological and behavioral variations,
both present and in the developmental future. Most of us check off the
"M" or the "F" box and choose the corresponding clothing, hair removal
routines, rest rooms, careers, urination positions, intimate partners, and
underarm deodorants.

Intersexuality—biologically variant sexuality—disturbs the conventional: both our institutional practices and our ways of thinking and
behaving. Though we are typically educated to think in binary terms,
there are common medical conditions that move human beings away
from the male and female norms. In this context it is useful to sketch and

explain some of the principle dimensions of "normality," both at the biological level (that is, sexuality) and the psychosocial level (that is, gender). We now sketch some complexities of sexual variation in the light of everyday concerns.

LOCKER-ROOM APPEARANCE

At the biological surface is what we look like in the locker room: male or female? While typical male and female genitalia (and breast development) represent the familiar bimodal distribution, there is a full spectrum in between.

EXTERNAL GENITALIA

The roots of sexual difference are to be found in embryology. It is a useful oversimplification to see baby girls as the default outcome of gestation, the developmental route that is taken unless androgenic hormones are present. For XY (male) embryos, a region on the Y chromosome induces the development of testes from undifferentiated gonadal tissue. The testes in turn produce virilizing androgens in sequences and quantities that can cause that which would otherwise become the labia majora to fuse into a scrotum, and cause that which would otherwise become the labia minora and clitoris to elongate and enlarge into a penis. In the absence of male hormones, which also inhibit feminization, the gonads become ovaries and the vagina and uterus develop.[39]

Apart from differences in size and shape, common visible anatomical variations for XY males include hypospadias, where the penis is open at some location other than at the end; bifid (divided) scrotum; and undescended testicles. Conversely, an XX female may have an enlarged clitoris, an absent or shallow vagina, partially fused labia, and so on.[40] In sum, external genitalia can be typically male, typically female, or virtually anywhere in between. A very large clitoris and a very small penis may be indistinguishable except for the term used to describe them.

FUNCTIONALITY

There are three principle dimensions in which function can be assessed. The first takes into account the *individual's ability to have sexual intercourse*. Is there a functional penis or vagina? A second dimension takes into account *erotic potential*. It is common for genital surgery to compromise erotic sensitivity and, to that extent, the intimate relationships that depend upon it. The third dimension considers *reproductive potential.* Is it possible to become a genetic and/or gestational mother or a genetic father?

GONADS

It is possible to have both ovarian and testicular tissues: true hermaphrodites by definition have both. Gonadal tissue may also be undeveloped in an adult (neither testicular nor ovarian), or it may develop anomalously (mixed gonadal dysgenesis). And gonadal tissue may be completely absent.[41]

ENDOCRINOLOGY

This dimension calls attention to hormone levels, their timing, and the body's responsiveness to them. Among many variations, two common ones can serve as examples. A condition called congenital adrenal hyperplasia (CAH) causes some XX fetuses to develop male-like external genitalia. Their adrenal glands produce large amounts of androgens, virilizing the fetus.[42] These children will sometimes menstruate through the phallus after puberty. A second condition called androgen insensitivity syndrome (AIS) causes XY fetuses to develop female external genitalia. Their testes produce androgens, but, because of a cellular abnormality that partially or completely inhibits response to the hormone, gestational development proceeds toward a female external morphology.[43]

GENETICS

In addition to the most common XX and XY karyotypes, there are also, for example, XO (Turner's syndrome, a sex chromosome missing), XXY (Klinefelter's syndrome), XYY, XXXY, XXYY or XXXYY. Embryos can also develop with XX cells in one part of the body and XY or other type cells in another part (mosaicism).[44]

CENTRAL NERVOUS SYSTEM

Hormones also organize the brain to bias an individual for future male-typical or female-typical behaviors. Laboratory experiments on mammals, for example, have elicited male behavior patterns in adult XX females after *in utero* exposure to androgens at critical stages of fetal development.[45] Likewise, female behavior patterns have been promoted in XY male mammals by prenatal exposure to anti-androgens.[46] Analogous phenomena have been observed with humans. This type of research supports the view that prenatal endocrinology biases psychosexual development by affecting the central nervous system. Rather than having been born neutral, the androgen-rich ambience in which John/Joan's brain developed probably accounts for her later masculine behavior and her suspicion, against the evidence, that she was really a boy.[47]

PSYCHOSOCIAL LIFE

While it remains to be seen how deeply our gendered behavior is neurologically hard-wired, there are at least three aspects of it that deserve consideration. The first calls attention to one's *sexual identity*. How does one see oneself at the deepest level? In addition to female and male, some now self-identify as intersexed. The second calls attention to one's *gender role*. How does one present publicly in dress, speech, gesture, and so on—as man or woman? And the third calls attention to *sexual orientation*. The condition of intersexuality precludes the application of terms like hetero- and homosexuality that conceive sexual desire, and its idealized object, in relation to the subject's sex. Instead, we reaffirm the recommendation to substitute the terms androphilic, gynecophilic, and ambiphilic.[48]

Because variation occurs independently at many of these levels, the total number of biological/psychosocial possibilities will be very large indeed. The study of intersexuality forces us far from the view that humanity comes in two mutually exclusive sexes, readily distinguishable at birth by the presence or absence of prominent external genitalia.

The discussion so far highlights four critical limitations in our capacity to manage intersexuality clinically. First, in the face of what to many is an astonishing variability, it appears impossible to draw any bright line that decisively and non-arbitrarily separates males and females. Second, even if there were such a procedure, parents lack the ability to engineer the psychosocial development of a target gender.[49] Third, we are unable to predict with confidence the gender that an intersexed newborn will settle into during adulthood. (Indeed, we are often enough mistaken even with anatomically typical infants.) And finally, given the deep and largely uncharted pervasiveness of the effects of being a typical male or female, it is unlikely that surgical reassignment will ever truly "normalize."

In the face of these four practical limitations, and the high probability that they will long endure, it may be time to accept that sex and gender have never been strictly binary; that, on the contrary, there have always been persons in between. In some cultures—various American Indian tribes and societies in Africa and New Guinea, for example—there are societal categories for persons who are neither men nor women

as we understand these terms.[50] Intersexuality is common and understandable. Rather than an occasion for emergency surgery and concealment, the birth of a baby with ambiguous genitalia may be an occasion
for medical, parental, and social humility and reflection, perhaps even
for celebration.

But, as Alice Dreger suggests,[51] the standard of practice represents
not humility at all, but a striking appropriation by doctors of the authority to use the arts of medicine to police the boundary between male and
female in the defense of cultural norms. Whether this *hubris* is inten-
tional or not, the surgical concealment of intersexuality lends support to
those who take for granted that there are but two sexual configurations,
each associated with a distinct gender and sexual preference. In making
available routine procedures for reconciling deviant anatomy to cultural
expectations, medicine vastly empowers the implementation of "normality" even, we would add, as it diminishes the value of difference.

Several commentators have observed the analogy between "normalizing" genital surgery and what has been called "female genital mutilation" as practiced on young girls in Islamic Africa. While both impose
morbidity and loss of function in the course of conforming a child's
genitalia to cultural expectations, medicine has been vocal in its condem-
nation of the latter, even as it continues to recommend the former. We
question whether physicians should ever sacrifice the organic functionality of any nonconsenting child—Somali or American—on the altar of
cultural expectation.

THREE RECOMMENDATIONS

FIRST RECOMMENDATION

*That there be a general moratorium on such surgery when it is done
without the consent of the patient.* In arriving at this first recommendation, we do not appeal to the premise that normalizing surgery in infancy does more harm than good. As noted earlier, the large-scale studies
that could confirm this are yet to be done. While only a skeptical premise
is warranted—that is, that we do not now know that surgery does more
good than harm—it suffices nonetheless to justify a moratorium.

As a firm rule, doctors should never undertake surgery, especially
without consent, unless there are disproportionate hazards associated
with all of the other options: Above all, do no harm. The presumption
has always to be against surgery unless two types of evidence are at hand.
First, one needs to know that comparable patients generally do well af-

ter the surgery: such data are not at hand regarding the adult beneficiaries of these surgeries. And second, one needs to know that comparable patients generally do badly without the surgery. Since surgery is always harmful per se, it should never be done unless there is an expectation of ample compensating benefits. Because this evidence is lacking, the surgical assignment of sex remains an experimental procedure: one in which the results cannot be properly assessed until at least 20 years after the intervention.

Accordingly, it is not possible for a patient's parents to give informed consent to these procedures, precisely because the medical profession has not systematically assessed what happens to the adults these infant patients become. Doctors can't tell parents what the long-term risks and benefits are because they haven't done the studies and don't know.

With the publication of the rest of the John/Joan story, and the additional research sketched above, the standard of practice appears to have lost the epistemic foundation it was earlier thought to have. And yet for some reason these operations continue, despite the erosion of their justification. We recommend that all pediatric surgical assignments be suspended until these issues are resolved.

Two caveats: We are not arguing that medically justified surgical interventions be withheld. Many conditions—bladder exstrophy, certain types of CAH—are associated with risks of morbidity, mortality, and loss of function. Such conditions should always be treated appropriately. And second, we are not suggesting that intersexed children be raised without gender. The choice of gender assignment should take into account the infant's condition, including its causes, and whatever is known about the prognosis.[52] The aim must be to raise infants in a way that will most probably turn out to be comfortable for the maturing child. But gender assignment has to be provisional, subject to revision by the intersexed child as he or she matures. Our objection is to the *surgical* assignment of sex, not to gender assignment per se.

SECOND RECOMMENDATION

That this moratorium not be lifted unless and until the medical profession completes comprehensive look-back studies and finds that the outcomes of past interventions have been positive. In part, this recommendation emerges from sympathy with the view that early surgery may be medically indicated for some types of intersexuality. We need to know more, for example, about the high incidence of cancer in cases of mixed gonadal dysgenesis.

But a stronger justification flows from medical integrity: the profession's ethical commitment to learn as much as it can, even when it makes mistakes.[53] Luckily, a 20-year double-blind prospective study is unnecessary. There are now many thousands of grown intersexuals who have and who have not had surgical and hormonal treatment. Retrospective outcome studies can now be done on these adults, uncovering the comparative effects of treatment and nontreatment. The willingness to subject its practices to honest scrutiny is part of what any profession owes to the community it serves, part of what makes the profession worthy of its community's trust.[54] Pediatrics has an obligation to assess the mature products of its handiwork.

Finally, these studies may be of significant benefit to intersexuals themselves. If the studies find these patients to be at risk for certain medical conditions, this information should be passed along so they can plan and act accordingly.

THIRD RECOMMENDATION

That efforts be made to undo the effects of past deception by physicians. For years, pediatric surgeons have stressed the necessity of rearing post-surgical intersexed infants as unambiguous boys or girls. We do not question that. However, in implementing this approach, parents and clinicians have often concealed aspects of surgery and treatment from the child and excluded maturing children from medical management decisions. Joan Hampson, one of Money's early co-authors, has remarked: "Oddly, even in children old enough to have some opinion, in our experience it has been rare that they have been given any opportunity to express it."[55] This practice can take the form of a well-intentioned, albeit deceptive, conspiracy between family and clinicians and against the child.

Taking the long view, one might ask when, if ever, these former patients should be told of their medical histories. Should it be the intention, at infancy, that these patients never be told or, rather, is the mature or maturing patient entitled to know? There is no standard that the pediatrician advise parents to disclose when their child reaches puberty or adulthood or at any other time. Adults who have had these procedures in childhood are now presenting at clinics, quite ignorant of their histories. This secrecy does damage to the patient. For success in deception entails that the adult patient not understand his or her medical condition. Just to the extent that these adults are misled, they cannot act rationally out of a realistic appraisal of their situation.

But a second objection proceeds from the observation that these cultivated illusions cannot be nurtured reliably and indefinitely. Often patients will discover their condition from an inadvertent family slip, community gossip, or personal investigation into puzzling aspects of their lives. As these children mature into full adulthood and initiate independent clinical relationships, the web of deception will weaken, at least to the extent that the patient develops genuine relationships of trust and confidence with doctors. Unless the entire profession is complicit (thereby ruling out genuine relationships of trust and confidence), one must expect that the truth will emerge. And when it does, the patient will learn, anyway, what she or he was never supposed to have found out. If the patient is going to find out anyway, surely it is better for the physician to initiate disclosure.

But even more disturbing than discovering the secret, the former patient will also discover that his or her deformity is unspeakably shameful in the minds of parents and physicians. Moreover, the former patient will learn that she or he has since childhood been systematically deceived by the very people who should have been the most trustworthy. These patients will often avoid physicians and become estranged from their parents. All of this is damaging. Most of it is needless. On a broader scale, it will not be only those patients who learn that physicians are willing to participate in deception. It will be the general community who come to know that doctors choreograph familial mendacity.

We recommend that the medical profession find ways to own up to these adults, initiating disclosure of the medical histories doctors have helped to conceal from their former pediatric patients. In addition to the ethical obligation, clinicians may even have legal duties to warn their former patients when matters of importance are discovered.[56]

One final conjecture. It may well be that this lack of candor is at the root of the profession's failure to do the needed outcome studies, the reason why so many former patients are "lost to follow up." For researchers cannot easily question former patients on the effects of surgery done in infancy when those same patients have never been informed of the surgery, let alone the reasons for it. Although our recommendations are threefold, they speak to a single complex problem. Parents cannot be informed of the expected outcome of the pediatric surgery because the adult outcome studies have not been done. And the adult outcome studies have not been done because these adults have not been informed of the surgery. We may have here an epistemological "black hole" that en-

traps parents, patients, and physicians in lies, secrets, and avoidable igno-
rance. While it will take intellectual integrity and professional courage
for these pediatric practitioners to extricate themselves, we expect the
profession will rise to this occasion.

ACKNOWLEGMENT

This work was supported by the Eugene Garfield Foundation, Philadelphia, and The Queens Medical Center Research Fund, Honolulu.
This chapter first appeared in *The Journal of Clinical Ethics* 9, no. 4 (Winter
1998): © 1998 by *The Journal of Clinical Ethics;* used with permission.

NOTES

1. J. Money and A.A. Ehrhardt, *Man and Woman, Boy and Girl* (Baltimore,
Md.: John Hopkins University Press, 1972).
2. The psychiatrist is quoted in J. Colapinto, "The True Story of John/
Joan," *Rolling Stone* (December 1997): 54-58, 60, 62, 64, 66, 68, 70, 72-73, 92, 94-
97.
3. J. Money, J.G. Hampson, and J.L. Hampson, "An Examination of Some
Basic Sexual Concepts: The Evidence of Human Hermaphroditism," *Bulletin of
the Johns Hopkins Hospital* 97 (1955): 301-19; J. Money, J.G. Hampson, and J.L.
Hampson, "Hermaphroditism: Recommendations Concerning Assignment of
Sex, Change of Sex and Psychological Management," *Bulletin of the Johns Hopkins Hospital* 97 (1955): 284-300.
4. S. Freud, *Three Essays on the Theory of Sexuality,* standard ed. 7 (London:
Hogarth Press, 1953, 1905); S. Freud, "Some Psychical Consequences of the
Anatomical Distinction between the Sexes," in *Collected Papers by Sigmund Freud,*
vol. 5, ed. J. Strachey (London: Hogarth Press, 1925).
5. Money and Ehrhardt, *Man and Woman,* see note 1 above; J. Money,
"Prenatal Hormones and Postnatal Socialization in Gender Identity Differentiation," *Nebraska Symposium on Motivation* 21 (1973): 221-95; J. Money, "Ablatio
Penis: Normal Male Infant Sex-Reassignment as a Girl," *Archives of Sexual Behavior* 4 (1975): 65-71.
6. Money, "Ablatio Penis," see note 5 above.
7. "Biological Imperatives," *Time,* 8 January 1973, 34.
8. E.A. Catlin and J.D. Crawford, "Neonatal Endocrinology," in *Principles
and Practice of Pediatrics,* 2d ed., ed. F.A. Oski et al. (Philadelphia, Penn.:
Lippincott, 1994), 421-29; P.K. Donahoe and J.J. Schnitzer, "Evaluation of the
Infant Who Has Ambiguous Genitalia, and Principles of Operative Management," *Seminars in Pediatric Surgery* 5 (1996): 30-40; M. Sifuentes, "Ambiguous
Genitalia," in *Pediatrics: A Primary Care Approach,* ed. C.D. Berkowitz (Philadelphia, Penn.: W.B. Saunders, 1996), 261-65.

9. R. Azziz et al., "Congenital Adrenal Hyperplasia: Long-Term Results Following Vaginal Reconstruction," *Fertility & Sterility* 46 (1986): 1011-14; P.K. Donahoe, D.M. Powell, and M.M. Lee, "Clinical Management of Intersex Abnormalities," *Current Problems in Surgery* 28 (1991): 517-79.

10. American Academy of Pediatrics, "Timing of Elective Surgery on the Genitalia of Male Children with Particular Reference to the Risks, Benefits, and Psychological Effects of Surgery and Anesthesia," *Pediatrics* 97 (1996): 590-94.

11. D. Cappon, C. Ezrin, and P. Lynes, "Psychosexual Identification (Psychogender) in the Intersexed," *Canadian Psychiatric Association Journal* 4 (1959): 90-106; M. Diamond, "A Critical Evaluation of the Ontogeny of Human Sexual Behavior," *Quarterly Review of Biology* 40 (1965): 147-75; M. Diamond, "Sexual Identity, Monozygotic Twins Reared in Discordant Sex Roles and a BBC Follow-Up," *Archives of Sexual Behavior* 11 (1982): 181-85; B. Zuger, "Gender Role Determination: A Critical Review or the Evidence from Hermaphroditism," *Psychosomatic Medicine* 32 (1970): 449-63.

12. S.J. Kessler, *Lessons from the Intersexed* (Piscataway, N.J.: Rutgers University Press, 1998).

13. H. Benjamin, *The Transsexual Phenomenon* (New York: Julian Press, 1966).

14. M. Blackless et al., "How Sexually Dimorphic Are We," *American Journal of Human Biology* (in press).

15. This estimate is by William Reiner, MD, quoted in Colapinto, "The True Story of John/Joan," see note 2 above.

16. Kessler, *Lessons from the Intersexed*, see note 12 above.

17. J.M. Schober, "Long-Term Outcome of Feminizing Genitoplasty for Intersex," in *Pediatric Surgery and Urology: Long-Term Outcomes*, ed. P.D.E. Mouriquand (Philadelphia, Penn.: W.B. Saunders, in press).

18. J. Money and M. Schwartz, "Biosocial Determinants of Gender Identity Differentiation and Development," in *Biological Determinants of Sexual Behavior*, ed. J.B. Hutchison (New York: John Wiley & Sons, 1978).

19. M. Diamond and H.K. Sigmundson, "Sex Reassignment at Birth: Long-Term Review and Clinical Implications," *Archives of Pediatrics and Adolescent Medicine* 151 (1997): 298-304.

20. Diamond, "Sexual Identity," see note 11 above.

21. Colapinto, "The True Story of John/Joan," see note 2 above.

22. Diamond and Sigmundson, "Sex Reassignment," see note 19 above.

23. Colapinto, "The True Story of John/Joan," see note 2 above; Diamond and Sigmundson, "Sex Reassignment," see note 19 above.

24. M.A. Mureau et al., "Satisfaction with Penile Appearance after Hypospadias Surgery: The Patient and Surgeon View," *Journal of Urology* 155 (1996): 703-6.

25. W.G. Reiner, "To Be Male or Female—That is the Question," *Archives of Pediatric and Adolescent Medicine* 151 (1997): 224-25.

26. William Reiner, MD, quoted in Colapinto, "The True Story of John/Joan," see note 2 above.

27. C. Chase, "Hermaphrodites with Attitude: Mapping the Emergence of Intersex Political Activism," *Gay & Lesbian Quarterly* 4 (1998): 189-211.

28. C.J. Dewhurst and R.R. Gordan, "Change of Sex," *Lancet* 309 (1963): 1213-17; M. Diamond, "Sexual Identity and Sexual Orientation in Children with Traumatized or Ambiguous Genitalia," *Journal of Sex Research* 34 (1997): 199-222; V. Khupisco, "The Tragic Boy Who Refuses to Be Turned into a Girl," *Sunday Times of Johannesburg* (21 May 1995): A-1.

29. K. Kipnis and G. Williamson, "Nontreatment Decisions for Severely Compromised Newborns," *Ethics* 95 (1984): 90-111.

30. J.M. Reilly and C.R.J. Woodhouse, "Small Penis and the Male Sexual Role," *Journal of Urology* 142 (1989): 569-72.

31. A.P. van Seters and A.K. Slob, "Mutually Gratifying Heterosexual Relationship with Micropenis of Husband," *Journal of Sex & Marital Therapy* 14 (1988): 98-107.

32. B. Craffey, "Showering 'Sans Penis'," *Chrysalis: The Journal of Transgressive Gender Identities* 2, no. 5 (Fall 1997/Winter 1998): 55-56.

33. Schober, "Long-Term Outcome," see note 17 above.

34. Kessler, *Lessons from the Intersexed*, see note 12 above.

35. J. Randolph, W. Hung, and M.C. Rathlev, "Clitoroplasty for Females Born with Ambiguous Genitalia: A Long-Term Study of 37 Patients," *Journal of Pediatric Surgery* 16 (1981): 882-87; A. Sotiropoulos et al., "Long-Term Assessment of Genital Reconstruction in Female Pseudohermaphrodites," *Journal of Urology* 115 (1976): 599-601.

36. Randolph, Hung, and Rathlev, "Clitoroplasty for Females," see note 35 above; T.M. Barrett, E.T. Gonzales, "Reconstruction of the Female External Genitalia," *Urologic Clinics of North America* 7 (1980): 455-63.

37. Kessler, *Lessons from the Intersexed*, see note 12 above.

38. Ibid., K.I. Glassberg, "The Intersex Infant: Early Gender Assignment and Surgical Reconstruction," *Journal of Pediatric and Adolescent Gynecology* 11 (1998): 151-54; J. Schober, "Early Feminizing Genitoplasty," *Journal of Pediatric and Adolescent Gynecology* 11 (1998): 154-56.

39. M. Diamond, "Human Sexual Development: Biological Foundation for Social Development," in *Human Sexuality in Four Perspectives*, ed. F.A. Beach (Baltimore, Md.: John Hopkins Press, 1976): 22-61.

40. M.M. Grumbach and F.A. Conte, "Disorders of Sex Differentiation," in *Williams Textbook of Endocrinology*, ed. J.D. Wilson et al. (Philadelphia, Penn.: W.B. Saunders, 1998), 1303-425.

41. Grumbach and Conte, "Disorders of Sex Differentiation," see note 40 above.

42. Ibid.

43. C. Quigley et al., "Androgen Receptor Defects: Historical, Clinical and Molecular Perspectives," *Endocrine Reviews* 16 (1995): 271-321.

44. C. Overzier, *Intersexuality* (New York: Academic Press, 1963).

45. C.H. Phoenix et al., "Organizing Action of Prenatally Administered Testosterone Propionate on the Tissues Mediating Mating Behavior in the Female Guinea Pig," *Endocrinology* 65 (1959): 369-82; R.W. Goy, J.E. Wolf, and S.G. Eisele, "Experimental Female Hermaphroditism in Rhesus Monkeys: Anatomical and Psychological Characteristics," in *Handbook of Sexology*, ed. J. Money and H. Musaph (Amsterdam, the Netherlands: Elsevier/North-Holland Biomedical Press, 1977), 139-56.

46. J. Vega-Matuszczyk and K. Larsson, "Sexual Preference and Feminine and Masculine Sexual Behavior of Male Rats Prenatally Exposed to Antiandrogen or Antiestrogen," *Hormones and Behavior* 29 (1995): 191-206.

47. Diamond, "Human Sexual Development," see note 39 above; M. Diamond, "Sexual Identity and Sex Roles," in *The Frontiers of Sex Research*, ed. V. Bullough (Buffalo, N.Y.: Prometheus, 1979), 33-56.

48. Diamond, "Sexual Identity," see note 28 above.

49. J.R. Harris, *The Nurture Assumption* (New York: Free Press, 1998).

50. R.B. Edgerton, "Poket Intersexuality: An East African Example of the Resolution of Sexual Incongruity," *American Anthropologist* 66 (1964): 1288-99; W.L. Williams, *The Spirit and the Flesh: Sexual Diversity in American Culture* (Boston: Beacon Press, 1986).

51. A.D. Dreger, *Hermaphrodites and the Medical Invention of Sex* (Cambridge, Mass.: Harvard University Press, 1998).

52. M. Diamond and H.K. Sigmundson, "Management of Intersexuality: Guidelines for Dealing with Persons with Ambiguous Genitalia," *Archives of Pediatrics and Adolescent Medicine* 151 (1997): 1046-50.

53. A.M Schwitalla, "The Real Meaning of Research and Why it Should Be Encouraged," *Modern Hospital* 33 (1929): 77-80; B. Barber, "The Ethics of Experimentation with Human Subjects," *Scientific American* 234 (1976): 25-31.

54. K. Kipnis, "Professional Responsibility and the Responsibility of Professions," in *Profits and Professions*, ed. W.L. Robison, M.S. Pritchard, and J. Ellin (Clifton, N.J.: Humana Press, 1983): 9-22.

55. J.G. Hampson, "Hermaphroditic Genital Appearance, Rearing and Eroticism in Hyperadrenocorticism," *Bulletin of the Johns Hopkins Hospital* 96 (1955): 265-73.

56. A.G. Nadel, "Duty of Medical Practitioner to Warn Patient of Subsequently Discovered Danger from Treatment Previously Given," *American Law Reports* 12, no. 4 (1981): 41.

18

A Mother's 10 Commandments to Medical Professionals: Treating Intersex in the Newborn

Helena Harmon-Smith

1. DO NOT tell the family to not name "the child"! Doing so only isolates them, and makes them begin to see their baby as an "abnormality."

2. DO encourage the family to call their child by a nickname (Honey, Cutie, Sweetie, or even "little one") or by a non-gender-specific name.

3. DO NOT refer to the patient as "the child." Doing so makes parents begin to see their child as an object, not a person.

4. DO call the patient by the nickname/name chosen by the parents. It may be uncomfortable at first but will help the parents greatly. Example: "How is your little sweetie doing today?"

5. DO NOT isolate the patient in an NICU [neonatal intensive care unit]. This scares the parents and makes them feel something is very wrong with their child. It isolates the family and prevents siblings, aunts, uncles and even grandparents from visiting and it starts a process within the family of treating the new member differently.

6. DO allow the patient to stay on a regular ward. Admit patients to the children's wing, perhaps in a single room. Then visitors are allowed, and bonding within the family can begin.

7. DO connect the family with an information or support group. There are many available: National Organization for Rare Disorders (NORD); Parent to Parent; HELP; AIS support group; Intersex Society of North America; even March of Dimes or Easter Seals.

8. DO NOT isolate the family from information or support. Do not assume they will not understand or will be more upset if they learn about other disorders or related problems. Let the parents decide what information they want or need. Encourage them to seek others out who can give them information and share experiences.

9. DO encourage the family to seek a counselor or therapist. Do not only refer them only to a genetic counselor; they will need emotional support as well as genetic information. Refer them to a family counselor, therapist, or social worker familiar with family crisis intervention/therapy.

10. DO NOT make drastic decisions in the first year. The parents need time to adjust to this individual child. They will need time to understand the condition and what their specific child needs. Allow them time to get over being presented with new information and ideas. Let them understand that their child is not a condition that must conform to a set schedule but an individual.

DO NOT schedule the first surgery before the patient even leaves the hospital. This will foster fear in the parents that this is life-threatening and that they have an abnormal or damaged child.

ACKNOWLEDGMENT

This list is from the website of the Hermaphrodite Education and Listening Post (HELP): < http://www.help@jaxnet.com >; © 1998 by Helena Harmon-Smith; used with permission.

19

Time for a Change

Heidi Walcutt

Until I learned about ISNA [the Intersex Society of North America] purely by chance at a talk in the spring of 1995 by Dr. Anne Fausto-Sterling, I had never spoken with anyone outside of Buffalo Children's Hospital about my intersexuality. I kept things to myself.

Questions. Problems. Shame.

I've spent my whole life with my feelings so bottled up. It's been really hard to change. I feel that it was my inability to talk about my problems that was a major cause of the breakup with my lover of two and a half years. No one ever told me what my diagnosis was when I was growing up.

I was raised as a girl, and first admitted to Buffalo Children's Hospital at age one in 1962. In 1966, surgeons there operated on my enlarged clitoris. In my recollection, it was a fully formed, functioning penis.

I have some clitoral sensation, and occasionally masturbate, but I am not sure whether I am orgasmic or not. I do experience some muscular contractions, though often I don't. I don't believe that anyone at Buffalo Children's ever spoke to me or asked me about genital sensation, orgasm, or masturbation, but it was a long time ago, and I can't say for sure.

No one explained anything to me before or immediately after the surgery, but at age 10 or 11 they began to bring me to Buffalo Children's for "counseling" sessions, about an hour long once per month. From age 15 to 17, the sessions were only about four times per year. In these sessions, I would sit with a psychologist for about an hour, and she would talk to me about very general concepts of being different. She told me that I was female, but my ovaries and uterus had been "underdeveloped," and that I would need to take pills prescribed by Buffalo physicians if I wanted to have puberty like other girls. Around age 14 or 15, they told me that I would need more surgery "if you ever want to have normal sex with your husband." Indeed, they scheduled the surgery, which was meant to increase the depth of my vagina, but it never happened. In any case I don't suppose that's very important, since I am entirely lesbian. But if I were interested in sex with men, I might feel differently, since the vagina they created during the first surgery is just a pocket, about half an inch deep, with flaps of skin on either side.

At age 17, they told me to take birth control pills, "to keep the hormones balanced in your system." They told me that, because of my unnamed "condition," I was similar to post-menopausal women, and that I might get weak bones if I didn't take the birth control pills. But the medications until then had put me on an emotional roller coaster, up one day and suicidally depressed the next. The psychologist never discussed this with me, but after a few months I just stopped taking them, and haven't taken them since. A little risk of weakened bones just didn't seem worth the pain of being back on that emotional roller coaster. [As Cheryl Chase has stressed, in fact there is a very high risk of early onset, severe osteoporosis for an intersexed individual whose gonads have been removed in childhood or adolescence by surgeons and who does not take replacement hormones. This risk is not really comparable to the risk of a post-menopausal woman. Early onset osteoporosis can be painful and debilitating in the extreme.—*Ed.*]

Dr. David Sandberg of Buffalo Children's Hospital has talked about the importance of long-term follow-up studies. But the hospital's idea of follow-up is laughable. They tracked me down once, when I was about 27, and asked me to come in for follow-up. I spent about an hour talking with a psychologist; that's it! "I'm a new psychologist, just getting started here, trying to find out how our former patients are doing," she told me.

At that time, at the age of 27, I was living with my parents. I had never been sexual with another person, mainly because I was still unable to accept that I was lesbian. I had never had the [secondary] vaginoplasty, and I had not taken hormones since age 17, in spite of the risk of osteoporosis. I was "coping" with my intersexuality by not coping with it, by simply squashing all my feelings. "How are you doing?" the psychologist asked me. "Fine," I told her. And I guess that's what she wrote down.

Dr. Sandberg says, "I cannot imagine anything worse than learning from a total stranger that all you had been told were lies or half-truths." I certainly wasn't told the truth at Buffalo as a patient. It was not until December of 1995 that I got the truth—that I had been diagnosed with gonadal dysgenesis, that surgeons at Buffalo Children's had removed my testes, and that all the staff there had conspired to lie to me, telling me that I was female but that my (nonexistent) ovaries and uterus were "underdeveloped."

The most important thing that I think could be done for intersex kids is to put together groups for them, so they can see that they aren't "the only one in the world." The counselors at Buffalo Children's Hospital told me that there were others, but they never let us meet. If there were a group, kids could talk about their feelings, about how they cope.

For instance, I remember "sex education" classes at school, around sixth grade. They separate the boys and girls, and talk about physical changes that "will happen to you," but nothing about sex itself. I knew I was different, that what I saw didn't apply to me, but I couldn't talk about this with my parents, who were conservative Christians, and I couldn't talk about it with the counselors at Buffalo Children's. The counselors just laid out for me what was going to happen to me, but I really couldn't talk about how I felt, or ask them questions. I was always uncomfortable in the counseling sessions, I would tell them almost anything so that I could just get out of there.

I remember, during high school, I read about hermaphrodites in Greek mythology and knew that it had to do with me, but I just locked it away deep in my mind, I couldn't discuss it. After all, who was I gonna talk to about that?! I couldn't talk to my Mom and Dad. There were the counselors at Buffalo Children's, but those sessions always followed the counselor's agenda. They would just explain what was going to happen to me.

Occasionally they would tell me, "We want to know what you're experiencing, what you're feeling." But there just wasn't a space there to talk about these kinds of things. They talked about "when you get married. . . . " I guess I could talk with these counselors more than with anybody else, but I just couldn't open up. I was sometimes suicidally depressed, especially with the hormone pills, but I just answered "fine" when they asked how I was.

I feel in between male and female. I don't really know what "masculine" feels like, but I don't feel like the "feminine" that I see in my Mom and my sisters, either. Because my family was so against homosexuality, I always tried to deny my lesbianism. I hoped to marry, adopt children, as the counselors at Buffalo Children's suggested. But I was never really attracted to men, and then I would see a girl, and feel this intense attraction.

Doctors should put together support groups for parents, so that they can talk about their experience with their intersex kids, know what to expect next, and get the encouraging feedback that they are not alone in dealing with this problem. My parents never spoke to me about my intersexuality, or about sex or sexuality in general. My Mom and I get along better now that I've moved three thousand miles away.

They shouldn't have these parades of interns, of surgeons, examining us and talking about us. A new physician wanting to learn about intersex should be interned to just one doctor, so that children will not have to be exposed to these big groups of students. Just one student, with one doctor.

I feel that they should encourage communication in the family, help them not to keep secrets. Kids are going to have questions, and they need to be told as much of the truth as they can handle at the time. As they get older and start to realize, "Hey, I'm different," they need honest explanations and the opportunity to decide what they want to do next.

It's wrong to rush the child off to surgery during infancy or early childhood because "everyone has to be either a boy or a girl"—but not intersexed. Surgery should be delayed until puberty, when the children can make decisions for themselves.

Of course, the only way children are going to be able to make these decisions and voice opinions is if they have been made to feel comfortable in dealing with these issues, and can trust the honesty and support of family and doctors.

ACKNOWLEDGMENT

An earlier version of this chapter was published as "Physically Screwed by Cultural Myth: The Story of a Buffalo Children's Hospital Survivor," in *Hermaphrodites with Attitude* (Fall-Winter 1995-1996): 10-11; © 1996 by ISNA; used with permission.

20

Take Charge!
A Guide to Home Auto-Catheterization

Sven Nicholson

I am now 44 years old. When I was 11, I had three operations to repair hypospadias. These operations were performed by a competent physician who considered my family a charity case and never sent us a bill. The artistry of his work has been commented on by most urologists who have subsequently examined me. He sincerely believed this was the best treatment for me, and did the best job he could. However, a stricture developed within two months of the final operation, and ever since my life has been drastically altered.

After these operations, my family moved. The next physician used a dilating procedure where a thin catheter was inserted, curling up inside the bladder, followed by a thicker catheter. Each increase in thickness required the lead catheter to curl up inside the bladder. It drove me crazy, but then we moved again, and the procedure used by the physician in the new neighborhood was worse.

He used steel probes to force the stricture open. The gruesome procedure had the same outcome every week: urine passed freely but painfully immediately after the procedure; then the stricture clammed up again a few hours later. Again and again my father had to drive me to the physician's home in the evening in order to open me up again. Though this physician was a professor at a research hospital, he never varied his technique or tried to solve the post-procedural problem.

Finally, I began to commute to a physician in another city who used a different set of catheters, made of rubber. Including the commute, the visits took about 10 hours, but the problem of "clamming up" did not recur, to my great relief.

Throughout my teenage years, physicians seemed to take the attitude that my condition could be somehow healed through a catheterization regime. In my early twenties, the physicians dropped this pretense. When I finished college, I became a lay missionary for my church. The mission board physician asked my urologist for a letter stating that my condition would not cause problems overseas. The physician gave me a set of silicon-coated catheters and instructed me in their use. His casual attitude reassured me, "You can live anywhere in the world, as long as there's soap and warm water." However, he was extremely reluctant to commit this to writing: in retrospect, I think that he did not want to create any written statement that a medical condition such as mine can be casually and easily treated by the patient himself. In any case, he wrote the letter (which I never saw) at the last minute and gave me a generous supply of anti-bacterial sulfa drugs and anesthetic lubricant, and I was on my way.

For several years I continued to visit physicians in order to receive prescriptions for anesthetic jelly and anti-bacterial sulfa drugs (gantrisin or gantinol) to protect against bladder infection while catheterizing myself. In my mid-thirties, I visited a urologist who refused to prescribe these drugs unless he first performed another surgery on me, to the tune of several thousand dollars. I determined to learn how to open my urethra without any prescription drugs.

I consider self-catheterization a vast improvement over visits to the urologist's office. The physician who gave me the catheters did so reluctantly, only because I was traveling overseas, and resisted making any kind of statement in writing about the ease with which this procedure could be performed by the patient himself. This reluctance probably has two sources; the first and obvious motivation is financial gain. The second is that any professional has seen amateurs botch things up, and naturally feels that s/he can do a better job. Regardless of the physician's attitude, I believe the patient is best served by obtaining his own set of catheters and treating himself.

I still use the set of silicon-coated catheters (sizes 14 to 24) I received before going overseas; they remain in perfectly good condition. The following paragraphs describe my "theory" and "method" of self-treatment, using this set of catheters.

LONG-TERM PROBLEMS

I catheterize myself about once a week. The urinary tract is normally sterile; though it involves no cutting, this is a surgical procedure performed at home, and I take it seriously. The problems encountered in treating urethral stricture by catheterization are: bladder infection; physical pain; various involuntary rejection reactions, including desire to urinate; and unnecessary stimulation of the prostate gland.

BLADDER INFECTION

The key is not drugs but simply to force fluids. On the day of catheterization I drink a lot of water and acidic fruit juices. On some occasions when I have been careless, I have developed an infection serious enough to cause fever, but cleared it out simply by forcing fluids.

A frequent desire to urinate may be a sign of bladder infection.

Another reason for forcing fluids is the soothing effect of passing a large amount of water soon after catheterization. This always makes me feel better. Diuretic teas, available in health food stores, help the body expel liquid by irritating the bladder. If you do develop a bladder infection, you may want to use these teas, but I think the irritation is a negative factor (this is true of caffeine, too).

To better understand the principle of forcing fluids to avoid bladder infection, envision bacteria: they like to live in colonies. A single bacterium by itself cannot produce enough chemicals to destroy the mucosal lining of the bladder, but a colony can do this. By constantly diluting the colony and the chemical they produce, you make it impossible for them to live and reproduce.

Water is really the best, being free of nutrients for the bacteria. Pure cranberry juice (almost undrinkably sour) is next, but it's difficult to obtain. Sweetened cranberry juice is useful, but contains lots of energy for the colonies you wish to destroy.

It is not advisable to insert the catheter all the way into the bladder. This is what causes bladder infections. As long as the widest part of the catheter is acting against the stricture, that's the main thing.

PHYSICAL PAIN;
INVOLUNTARY REJECTION REACTIONS;
UNNECESSARY STIMULATION OF PROSTATE

I don't understand these completely, but they are all factors that I consider in living my life and developing my procedure. There are psychological links between physical pain and stimulation of the prostate, but I don't think in "psychosomatic" terms. Rather, I have noticed that my urethra has a mind of its own, and I need to pay attention. Sometimes it wants to clam up, to prevent the introduction to any catheter. At other times it's yielding. Sometimes it get inflamed, even angry. I don't think of it as a "voice" that I must "listen" to, but over the years I've developed some ideas about what it wants and what makes it happy. Similarly, my bladder and my prostate also have their own ideas about the things that get done to them.

Basically my approach is to reduce stress and make the experience as pleasant as possible for everybody.

MY PROCEDURE

If I have gone, say, two or three weeks without catheterization and I know my urethra is getting tight, I will be especially careful to use over-the-counter analgesics such as aspirin, Tylenol, and Ibuprofen 20 minutes before catheterization (sometimes I use all three; I've never checked if this actually increases effectiveness or not). I do not use wine or marijuana because these drugs throw the judgment off.

Alcoholic beverages deaden the sense of touch. Under the influence of alcohol, I might force the catheter in roughly, only to feel the effects later on. Caffeine enhances the effect of aspirin, but it also makes the hands jumpy and irritates the bladder. This might cause a "spastic" desire to urinate later on. (The effect is slight; I usually have coffee every day whether I plan on therapy or not.)

RELAXING ATMOSPHERE

At first I simply sat on the commode and treated myself, but this is an extremely uncomfortable position for catheterization and psychologically reinforces the inherent ugliness of the act.

It's far better to think of catheterization as one type of personal grooming. I like to shave when I'm taking a bath or shower. My skin is more relaxed and cooperative, and I seem to be able to shave an extra millimeter or two off each whisker. I recommend that catheterization be integrated into the bathing routine. In detective novels, one sometimes reads about someone who slashed their wrists in the bathtub. The reason? The hot water deadens the pain.

I rate locations as follows: (1) hot bath; (2) hot shower; (3) in bed while, for example, reading an absorbing book. Warmth during and after the operation are essential. During the winter, plan on staying indoors afterwards.

I have noticed that if a "spastic" desire to urinate occurs, it usually happens during cold or chilly weather.

CHOICE OF SALVE

After forsaking prescription drugs, I first used KY jelly. Then medicated jellies began to appear in the drug stores for males who had difficulty maintaining an erection during coitus. The jelly works by deadening the penis. This is an inexpensive way to treat the immediate pain. Medicated jellies might not be available over-the-counter in foreign countries, so bring extra tubes when you travel. In an emergency, you might use almost any household oil to lubricate the catheter, even butter or olive oil. However, the oil will heat up due to friction when the catheter is introduced, so in this case, you must be extra slow.

Some commercial brands of medicated jellies are Detain and Maintain. The Maintain label says: "desensitizing lubricant for men. Active Ingredient: Benzocaine 7.5% in a water washable base. Also contains carbomer, Polyethylene Glycol." The carrier jelly itself is water soluble, but one of the other ingredients seems to be insoluble in water and soap. I find this ingredient slightly irritating and I hope I never develop an allergy to it, because it would be hard to live without it.

The insoluble ingredient seems to cling to the skin, and the urethra produces a mucous to wash it out; this process takes a little over 24 hours, during which time mucous will likely come in contact with the scrotum and adjacent areas. For this reason, plan to change underwear after the operation (say, four to six hours later), and take a shower before you go to bed. Although the ingredient doesn't seem to be water- or soap-soluble, it does respond to washing; perhaps it is the mechanics of sluicing water.

CATHETERIZATION

When I was visiting physicians during my teenage years, a major emphasis was placed on dilation up to 24 Foley. I'm not sure that my masculinity depends on the internal diameter of my urethra; in terms of plumbing, anything above about 14 is fine.

I prefer to perform the operation in the bathtub. Immediately prior to inserting a catheter, I wash it with warm water and mild soap (for example, "Dove"; I'm allergic to stronger soaps). I also wash the area around the genitals more than once. Sometimes I hold the catheter in my teeth while I wash my genitals (so it doesn't have to touch anything); in this case, I hold the "distal" end (not the end to be inserted).

I usually begin catheterization by applying the medicated jelly to a 14 catheter and introducing this to deaden the tissue in the urethra. At the same time, I apply it to the outside of the penis; the chemical seems to penetrate through the tissue. The purpose is to make the tissue numb, not to widen the stricture. Then I wash my hair. Then rinse. Now the urethra is numb. Then I wash the 16 catheter and coat it with jelly. While that's inside, I might shave or use a pumice stone to remove dead skin from my feet.

You get the idea. Because I'm scrubbing my back, stimulating my scalp, and tending my toes, my mind is not focused on the area of the operation, except at those moments when I'm actually inserting a catheter. I don't go beyond 18. Catheterization is a type of personal grooming. I expect as much pain and pleasure from it as I do from shaving or brushing my teeth.

I keep the water as hot as the water heater will let me. When I'm done, I run the shower for a bit to sluice off the irritating "active ingredient."

Usually, I don't actively remove the catheters. The urethra seems to expel them naturally while I'm washing other parts of my body. (Or, the effect of gentle washing movements is to cause the catheter to be expelled.) I often leave the bathtub without removing the final catheter.

POST-OP

After the operation, I always plan on doing something sedentary: respond to e-mail, read, have a meal with a friend. I can circumspectly leave the catheter in for these activities. I think leaving the catheter in for a longer period of time increases the effectiveness of the operations. The urethra seems to have a mind of its own, sometimes tightening around the catheter, sometimes relaxing and allowing it to drop out. Promote relaxation. Usually, the catheter will be expelled within 30 minutes, depending on my level of activity.

I usually have something hot to drink right away, preferably an herbal tea (but not diuretic). The main thing is the fluid, and secondarily the relaxation. Some teas, such as echinacea, stimulate the immune system and thus have a positive effect in preventing bladder infection. Obviously, there is no reason why you can't have alcoholic beverages at this time, if you so choose. The major consideration is not the type of beverage, but the amount. A large Evian Spring Water bottle contains 1.5 liters of water. Try to drink two. Passing large quantities of water has a soothing effect, both psychologically, physically, and chemically (it helps to expel the irritant in the salve).

Your physician has probably already given you a list of activities which should be avoided; riding bicycles, equestrian sports, sliding down banisters, and so on.

REFLECTIONS

As I mentioned earlier, the surgeon who treated me did not charge for his services. I'm sure he sincerely felt that this was the best course of action for me. In retrospect, I wish that the operations had never happened, that I had simply been allowed to live out my life with the plumbing system originally given to me by my Creator.

The operation was explained briefly to me at the outset, but alternatives were never discussed, no scenario other than the desired outcome was ever presented. I had never heard of "informed consent," and it would not have applied to my situation.

The hypospadias repair was performed in three stages, when I was eleven years old. Between the ages of 12 and 16, I lived a life of denial alternating with acute crises. Under the care of one physician, a urology professor at a medical university, my urethra would actually become completely occluded after dilation, rather than become more open. Yet he never varied his procedure in the slightest way, which suggests that he also continued teaching his students the same counter-productive methods. So much for research hospitals.

During my high school years, while all this was happening, popular culture was full of references to Freud, to counselors and therapists and psychoanalysts and pastors who had a counseling ministry, et cetera, et cetera. Yet none of this affected my life. Not once did I discuss my problem with a trained counselor. Nor did my parents. And probably my doctors never looked at the problem in psychological terms.

No literature existed. I was encouraged to deny reality, to think that the cure lay in just a few more visits to the doctor.

I've never heard of a contest where men parade the internal diameters of their urethras, and I'm not sure how it would be done. However awkward the concept might be, much of the therapy I received for the first 10 years seems to have been designed with the intention to prepare me to become a world champion.

When I started treating myself, my first act was to abandon this concept. Which is not to say that I stopped denying reality. But my weird world is more comfortable to live in now. I open my urethra just as far as necessary to allow me to pass urine.

I'm sure I'll have more problems as I grow older, but I don't know what they will be, and I suspect that doctors don't understand them either. In any case, I have no desire to become a world champion in a masculine beauty contest—a ticker tape parade down Fifth Avenue, as the challengers for widest urethra in the welterweight division for 65-year-old and older head toward Madison Square Garden.

ACKNOWLEDGMENT

This chapter first appeared in *Chrysalis: The Journal of Transgressive Gender Identities* 2, no. 5 (Fall 1997/Winter 1998); © 1998 by Sven Nicholson; used with permission.

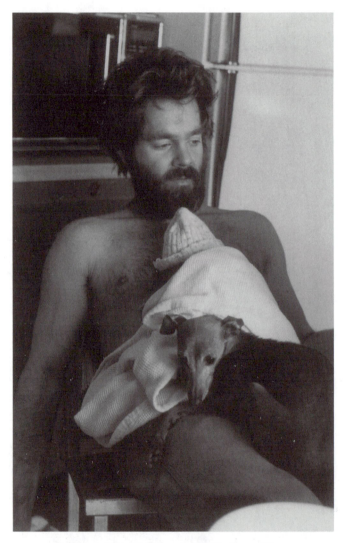

Edmund G. Howe and Chelsea Howe

21

Intersexuality:
What Should Careproviders Do Now?

Edmund G. Howe

The authors in this book ask how intersexuals should be medically treated, based on what we know now.[1] They urge, above all else, that surgeons no longer operate on infants born with ambiguous genitals to create "more normal looking" genitals. To answer the question of whether this surgery should be done, it is necessary to answer several more far-reaching questions, some of which strike to the core of who, as humans, we are. How, for instance, do we acquire our sexual identity? Is it through nature or nurture? Can parents' love protect their children from the harmful effects of social stigma? If it can, can parents overcome any prejudice they may have acquired so that they can provide this love, and how can they accomplish this? Can persons have fulfilling intimate sexual relationships if they have ambiguous genitals?

In this essay I will explore what careproviders should do now. On another tack, I will suggest that intersexual persons tend to have exceptional insight; I discuss what this insight is, and indicate why it has universal relevance.

THE BASES OF THE CONTROVERSY

Surgeons reconstruct children's ambiguous genitals because they believe that early surgery is necessary for two reasons: (1) to enable children to acquire an intact sexual identity, and (2) to enable parents to sufficiently overcome any ambivalence they feel, so that they can give their children the love they need. Surgeons believe that the brain is sufficiently "plastic" that if they restructure these infants' genitals, their sexual identity will follow suit. They assume that sexual identity is formed by nurture, not nature—by parents raising children as one or the other gender, rather than by genes or prenatal hormones.

Some of those who oppose the performance of surgery on intersexual infants, including many intersexuals themselves, do so in large part because many who have had this surgery report that they subsequently acquired a gender identity that is different from their anatomically assigned gender. They believe that if surgery should be done at all, it should be done much later, when children have acquired a permanent identity and can consent.

Many of those who have had surgery also argue against it because of its psychological effects. They report that surgery made them feel ashamed, as if there were something profoundly wrong with them. They report that this feeling of shame was exacerbated by large numbers of doctors coming to their hospital bedside to view their genitals.

These individuals report that this shame was further exacerbated by doctors withholding information, which implied that their condition was too shameful to discuss.[2] Others who have had this surgery, finally, report that they have less sensation in their genital area and even feel pain. They contend that if they had not had surgery, they could form just as meaningful intimate sexual relationships and enjoy sexual sensations that would not have been diminished.

WHY IS THIS CONTROVERSY
SO HEATED?

The parties in this discussion have become increasingly estranged. Alice Domurat Dreger, who compiled the writings in this volume, informs us that she invited some of those who have acted as proponents of infant surgery to present their arguments, but none accepted.[3] Intersex activist Cheryl Chase reports that, when a clinician presented data at a conference that appeared to be critical of early surgery, his colleagues "turned on [him] like vicious dogs."[4] Sociologist Sharon Preves reports that even some intersexual persons consider those who are politically active in opposing infant surgery to be "radical."[5]

It is important to recognize the issues that may contribute to this controversy and impede its resolution. Careproviders have a responsibility to hear patients' views and discuss them, and patients have a responsibility to raise opposing views respectfully. Additionally, it may be necessary, as Crouch implies, for careproviders and intersexuals to band together to effect the "positive clinical and cultural change" that he believes is needed.[6] I will argue that trust between patients and careproviders may be more important to intersexuals' welfare than any other goal that is immediately achievable.

From the surgeons' standpoint, critics of infant surgery may not represent those who have benefited most from it. These surgeons believe that critics fail to recognize this possibility, and fail to recognize how badly they—and others—might have fared if they had not had surgery. Further, these surgeons believe that critics may be unhappy for other reasons, such as the difficulties their conditions impose, and that they blame their unhappiness on surgery, because it serves exceptionally well as a scapegoat.[7] The complexity of these issues is evidenced in that each of these suppositions is psychologically plausible: persons who feel shame find it more difficult to appreciate others' points of view.[8]

If this psychological possibility has any validity at all, however, it paradoxically supports what critics of surgery have argued: that early, unconsented surgery shouldn't be done. Clearly, clinicians' first goal is to help intersexual infants have positive psychological outcomes. If the reason that intersexuals oppose early surgery is that they have experienced such shame that they cannot feel empathy, avoiding this outcome should prevail over any other!

In the view of critics, surgeons may have first performed infant surgery on the basis of unsubstantiated theory and, thereafter, have over-relied on medical authorities to justify it.[9] More recently, surgeons have been criticized because they have not accorded enough weight to patients' reports of adverse outcomes. There is a psychological reason that careproviders may ignore reports of adverse outcomes: if the claims are true, surgeons would have to acknowledge that performing surgery was a mistake. This would be exceedingly painful. The only way to avoid this pain would be to deny that these claims are true.

WHAT SHOULD
CAREPROVIDERS DO NOW?

All this having been said, I believe that surgeons have acted in good faith in the past; as Preves writes, "I believe that these 'sexing' procedures are motivated by a sincere desire to assist intersexuals and their families in achieving social acceptance."[10] I believe that the disagreement stems mostly from a mutually exclusive empirical view. Which view is correct may be impossible to discern.[11] What, then, should careproviders do?

The pros and cons of performing infant surgery may vary with the intersexual condition.[12] After careful review, it may be found that there is no compelling proof that surgery should be performed for most conditions. If so, this is neither surprising, nor grounds for attributing blame—after all, only 15 to 20 percent of medical practices now carried out have been shown to be justified, based on "rigorous scientific" studies.[13]

Deciding what to do must begin with recognizing the one goal that is most important for intersexuals, and both surgeons and those who oppose surgery agree on this: for these children, as they grow up, to be happy.

This priority is the right one. It is well-acknowledged that how patients perceive their disorders affects them much more profoundly than what their disorders actually are. Even the activist Chase, who adamantly opposes early surgery and who is an intersexual, states, "The primary source of harm . . . is not surgery per se but the [shameful] attitude."[14] In regard to this goal, current approaches appear to have failed: one study of intersexuals by Slipjer and colleagues reports that the percentage of intersexuals who have "general psychopathology" is *39 percent.*[15]

Can anything be done to attempt to reduce this percentage? Two new approaches might be considered. Both involve the possibility that intersexuals' emotional problems are, to a significant degree, the product of their surgeons' suggestion: that surgeons have insisted on early surgery suggests to both intersexuals and their parents that the condition is a source of shame. Chase states, "Early surgery is one means by which that message is conveyed to parents and to intersexed children."[16] Parents reinforce this message as their children grow, as well. Probably the one most important factor that enables children to withstand and transcend social stigma so that they can grow up and be healthy is having self-esteem. This quality results mostly from having parents who unconditionally love and accept them.[17]

Unfortunately, it appears that current approaches fail to help parents to unconditionally love and accept their intersex children, according to Slipjer and colleagues. The percentage of parents "not able to work through the trials and tribulations their child's lack of gender clarity entailed" was *50 percent.*[18]

As already stated, when surgeons recommend surgery in infancy, it may induce feelings of shame in the parents toward their child. This psychological effect is identified in Harmon-Smith's "A Mother's 10 Commandments to Medical Professionals: Treating Intersex in the Newborn," when she states that scheduling the first surgery before the child leaves the hospital can "foster fear in the parents that . . . they have an *abnormal and damaged* child" [italic added].[19] If this is a source of shame, what else can be done?

REGARDING INFANT SURGERY
AS DISCRETIONARY

If surgery could be postponed or not done at all, careproviders could present parents with various views, rather than stating that surgery should be done.[20] They might help parents to contact persons with alternative views, like the authors of the chapters of this book. Further, "impartial persons," such as ethics consultants, might help parents work these views through.

Careproviders could treat intersexuals as they (until recently) treated patients with Parkinson's disease. (Parkinson's differs, of course, from intersex in two respects: first, Parkinson's is a pathology, whereas many argue that intersex is merely a variation in anatomy; second, in the case of Parkinson's, it is the patient who consents.) Some Parkinson's patients have abnormal movements that no longer respond to medication (this is the reason there is the need—for those who accept the procedure—to have fetal tissue transplants). Until recently, brain surgery could reduce these movements, but only at a dear cost: if the surgeon's knife went "too far," it could cut too many of the wrong kind of nerve connections, and could cause *greater* abnormal movements.[21] Surgeons would routinely discuss the risks and benefits of this procedure, and patients would decide. Allowing patients to decide fostered trust and involved no shame.

REGARDING SURGERY
AS RESEARCH

This is analogous to the approach that careproviders take when helping patients decide whether to enter a research protocol. In this instance, careproviders *cannot* favor one choice over another, because, if clinical equipoise truly exists, it is not possible to know whether a subject will benefit from the protocol or not. Since parents cannot know whether their intersexed child will benefit more from having surgery or not, therapeutic research may not be merely a metaphor for this surgery, but may, in fact, be the truth. (This presupposes, of course, that this surgery is therapeutic, when, in fact, it may be cosmetic and unwarranted altogether.)

REGARDING PARENTS' AMBIVALENCE AS PATHOLOGICAL

Another intervention careproviders may wish to consider goes a step further. They could tell parents that if they feel ambivalence toward their infant that prevents them from loving the infant as they truly want to, this ambivalence is a pathological response, and they should seek therapy.

This assessment may be true. If parents respond to their own ambivalence by avoiding their child, the behavior is phobic. If they have thoughts about their child that interfere with loving the infant, the thoughts are obsessional. Phobic behavior and obsessional thoughts can be treated.[22] Further, even if parents who have these responses don't seek therapy, that a careprovider has made such a recommendation communicates unequivocally that they should not feel shame.

It may be, of course, that early surgery, in its net effect, may be beneficial for some children, but harmful for others: after all, individuals differ greatly in the degree to which they are susceptible to suggestion (in this case, the degree to which early surgery would induce feelings of shame). But those individuals who are more susceptible to experiencing shame would be the same individuals who would be most severely emotionally impaired by receiving early surgery. As this is the case, careproviders should not do surgery, in order to avoid inducing this shame.

HELPING THESE CHILDREN RESPECT THEMSELVES IN OTHER WAYS

Careproviders may employ numerous interventions to help intersexual children. The authors in this book discuss many of them, such as not examining intersexuals' genitals before groups and helping intersexuals to "connect with" others having the same disorder. Counseling may be helpful, yet the maximal approaches for helping these children remain to be developed.

Approaches developed for homosexuals are designed to help them through the different crises they are likely to experience in their lives. In early adolescence, for instance, they may come out too soon to "rebel," and this may increase their problems. In mid-adolescence, they may stay too close to their parents due to fear that their peers will reject them. In late adolescence they may avoid pursuing intimate partners because they fear these partners will reject them. This last avoidance response may be particularly self-destructive. To avoid this intimacy, they may project the unresolved homophobia they feel toward themselves to others to whom they feel attracted. Each time they do this, their contempt for themselves may increase.[23]

Intersexual persons may also be prone to having each of the above responses. The counseling they receive must obviously differ from that of homosexuals. They will need counseling from a much earlier age, and the counseling they are provided must be tailored and progressively altered, according to their age. This tailoring is also necessary in deciding not only what information to give, but how. If information given is not titrated according to age, the information may be harmful.

One counselor writes: "Whereas at one time it was customary to withhold discussing information until a child was old enough to understand it, it is now recognized as more helpful to tell the truth stage by stage as understanding unfolds."[24] She illustrates this approach with the case of a child with androgen insensitivity syndrome (AIS).[25] When, if ever, should girls with AIS—who are in all relevant respects female—be told that they have a Y chromosome (the usual marker for male gender)? The counselor points out that, between ages two and six, it is not necessary to provide much information, because children of this age usually don't make "superficially disparaging comparisons." At age 12, on the other hand, children can comprehend adult language. The counselor reports that she told a 12 year old with AIS that all embryos are, in fact, initially girls; and, that thus, the building blocks that enabled her to grow merely had XY on them as a label. The counselor then showed the child a film of a mother with AIS happily raising two adopted children.[26]

CAN INTERSEXUALS HAVE EQUALLY FULFILLING, INTIMATE SEXUAL RELATIONSHIPS WITHOUT SURGERY?

Some intersexuals who have had surgery contend that surgery to amend ambiguous genitals should never be performed without the consent of the person at risk. Whether surgery is ever desirable may depend on the extent to which persons without surgery have wholly fulfilling sexual intimacy with their partners. This answer may be unknown, but some new findings regarding the sensory potential of persons who have had nerve injuries may warrant consideration.

First, surgical techniques have improved over time,[27] although, as Chase notes, this surgery still may cause decreased sensitivity and pain,[28] and the degree to which it does will not be known for years. Second, it is possible that persons who have had this surgery may be able to increase their sexual responsivity by providing greater stimulation to the nerve pathways that remain.

For example, it was assumed until recently that patients who had complete spinal cord injuries (SCI) could not experience sexual pleasure from being stimulated below their injury. Now it is known that this is not true, most likely because nerves outside the spinal cord carry sexually stimulating impulses to the brain.[29] As many as *52 percent* of female patients with SCI have been able to experience orgasm utilizing various techniques, which include the use of a vibrator, or asking a partner to stimulate them for a longer period of time.[30] Although the nerves that are injured in SCI are different from those damaged by surgeries performed on many intersexuals, these techniques could enhance intersexuals' sexual pleasure. A second recent and unexpected neurological finding is that when persons lose sexual sensation in one part of their body, sensation may increase in another part.[31] This increased sensitivity seems to be due to a compensatory response, in which nerves grow or "sprout" in a new part of the body when they have been damaged in another.[32]

The data from these studies, which indicate that lost sensitivity may be compensated by new sensitivity, may be used to continue the justification of early surgery on intersexual infants. The same data may be used more powerfully, however, to argue the opposite: we know that persons who have SCI have been successful in increasing their sexual responsivity by asking a partner to stimulate them for a longer time or to stimulate other parts of their body; if loving partners will help in these ways, surely there are loving partners who would be as willing to interact sexually with intersexuals who have not had surgery, especially since these individuals would be more normally, easily, and intensely aroused.

CONCLUSION

Surgeons are right when they state that the brain is incredibly plastic. This insight, however, may be misapplied; as just described, the brain can create sexual responsivity in degrees and in places it has not been before. This same plasticity may enable parents who initially have negative responses toward an intersexual infant to overcome these responses so that they can give their child the love their child needs.

Intersexual persons may model, more than any other group, how the brain's plasticity may "prevail." Those who have succeeded in acquiring meaningful intimate relationships have, after all, had a unique and exceedingly difficult interpersonal experience. They have had to disclose that they are intersexual and then work through whatever feelings this engenders.

It is curious and even intriguing that throughout the ages and in different cultures, intersexual persons have been viewed as having exceptional insight.[33] If there is any truth to this claim, some might postulate it has to do with their experiencing exceptional hormones or having lived through the experience of being each sex. One man who had been raised as a girl believed he had unusual and greater insight, because he had experienced what it felt like "from both sides."[34] It is possible, however, that intersexuals simply have unique interpersonal difficulties, and, if they can transcend them, they may acquire an insight that most other persons lack.[35]

What is the nature of this insight? This question is best answered in presenting the words of a person who has this insight, who underwent sexual reassignment as a child. "John," a 31-year-old man, suffered the complete loss of his penis due to a "botched circumcision when he was 8 months old."[36] Operations were performed to feminize his appearance, "followed by a 12-year program of social, mental and hormonal conditioning to make the transformation take hold in his psyche." On orders from his doctor, he was given no information regarding the reason for his continuing surgery, routine cross-country trips to have extensive genital exams, and hormonal treatment. On reaching puberty, John (renamed "Joan"), told his mother that he would kill himself if he was again forced to see the doctor who performed the lengthy exams. His mother supported him, and, shortly after, John "simply stopped living as a girl." He later had surgery and hormonal treatment to try to restore his masculine appearance, and his father gave him his complete medical history, including the reasons for his parents' actions.

John eventually married a woman who had three children. When asked what he would say to the doctor most responsible for his ordeal, he acknowledged that his fantasies once had been violent. Now, he says, "What's done is done."

This capacity for forgiving is another aspect of the brain's plasticity. When asked how he would regard the role of being a husband and father, he demonstrated the exceptional insight that intersexuals may tend to have: he replied that there's " 'much more to being a man than just *bang bang bang* sex. . . . You treat your wife well. . . . You're a good father. . . . That, to me, is a man.' "

ACKNOWLEDGMENT

This chapter first appeared in *The Journal of Clinical Ethics* 9, no. 4 (Winter 1998); © 1998 by *The Journal of Clinical Ethics*; used with permission. Photo used with the permission of Chelsea Howe.

NOTES

1. Throughout this introduction, I do not refer to intersexuals as "patients" because, as some intersexuals claim, their condition may not be justifiably regarded as a disorder. In regard to whether intersexuals should be regarded as having a psychiatric disorder, see H.F.L. Meyer-Bahlburg, "Intersexuality and the Diagnosis of Gender Identity Disorder," *Archives of Sexual Behavior* 23, no. 1 (1994): 21-40.

2. Ironically, shame may be greatest in those children who have had the *most* nurturing parents. This may be because these children, having received more love, acquire greater expectations for themselves. See J. Belsky, C. Domitrovich, and K. Crnic, "Temperament and Parenting Antecedents of Individual Differences in Three-year Old Boys' Pride and Shame Reactions," *Child Development* 68, no. 3 (June 1997): 456-66.

3. Dreger invited, among others, John Money of Johns Hopkins University, who declined.

This response may be not be uncommon. As another example, John Gearhart, a "pro-surgery advocate . . . always refused to engage in a dialogue with intersex activists." D. Romesburg and Gay and Lesbian Alliance Against Defamation, "Intersex People Hidden Behind Potted Plants," *Hermaphrodites with Attitude* (Fall 1997): 2.

4. C. Chase, "Surgical Progress Is Not the Answer to Intersexuality," chapter 15 of this book.

5. S.E. Preves, "For the Sake of the Children: Destigmatizing Intersexuality," chapter 4 of this book.

6. R.A. Crouch, "Betwixt and Between: The Past and Future of Intersexuality," chapter 3 of this book.

7. See Preves's comments on the difficulty of making conclusions about *all* intersexual persons. She conducted 41 in-depth interviews in an attempt to find a representative sample. Preves, "For the Sake of the Children," see note 5 above.

8. Patients under stress may, for example, experience increased pain in areas in which they have had surgery. Not knowing that this process is taking place, they may blame this pain solely on the surgery. R.A. Sherman, C.J. Sherman,

and G.M. Bruno, "Psychological Factors Influencing Chronic Phantom Limb Pain: An Analysis of the Literature," *Pain* 28 (1987): 285-95.

9. K.P. Leith and R.F. Baumeister, "Empathy, Shame, Guilt, and Narratives of Interpersonal Conflicts: Guilt-Prone People are Better at Perspective Taking," *Journal of Personality* 66, no. 1 (February 1998): 28.

10. Preves, "For the Sake of the Children," see note 5 above.

11. "It must be emphasized that this patient population needs to be assessed in careful longitudinal studies." W.G. Reiner, "Sex Assignment in the Neonate with Intersex or Inadequate Genitalia," *Archives of Pediatric and Adolescent Medicine* 151 (October 1997): 1044-45, at 1045.

12. M.R. Zaontz and M.G. Packer, "Abnormalities of the External Genitalia," *Pediatric Urology* 44, no. 5 (October 1997): 1267-97.

13. J.Z. Ayanian et al., "Rating the Appropriateness of Coronary Angiography: Do Practicing Physicians Agree with an Expert Panel and with Each Other?" *New England Journal of Medicine* 338, no. 26 (June 1998): 1896-904; P.G. Shekelle et al., "The Reproducibility of a Method to Identify the Overuse and Underuse of Medical Procedures," *New England Journal of Medicine* 338, no. 26 (June 1998): 1888-95.

14. Chase, "Surgical Progress," see note 4 above.

15. F.M.E. Slijper et al.,"Long-Term Psychological Evaluation of Intersex Children," *Archives of Sexual Behavior* 22, no. 2 (1998): 125-44.

16. Chase, "Surgical Progress," see note 4 above.

17. "The family is seen as being a particularly powerful source of self-esteem related values that can have a greater impact than general forces." E.B. Katz, "Self-Esteem: The Past of an Illusion," *American Journal of Psychoanalysis* 58, no. 3 (1998):303-15, at 311, citing C. Mruk, *Self-Esteem: Research, Theory and Practice* (New York: Springer, 1995), 64.

18. Slijper et al., "Long-Term Psychological Evaluation," see note 15 above. Parents may be unable to transcend their initial response when infants are born with other "defects" as well. I think, for example, of my first psychiatric patient. She became blind when she had received too much oxygen in her incubator. Her parents remained in love with each other and neither remarried, but they were unable to overcome their feelings after their child was blinded and obtained a divorce.

19. H. Harmon-Smith, "A Mother's 10 Commandments to Medical Professionals: Treating Intersex in the Newborn," chapter 18 of this book.

20. Hurtig states, "The development of gender identity appears to be an intricate interaction of hormonal forces and rearing practices. . . . The goal of the clinician is *not* to unilaterally make life-shaping decisions, but to help the patient or the parent to express and understand the nature of their ambivalence in order to reach workable [sic] resolution of their dilemma." A.L. Hurtig, "The Psychosocial Effects of Ambiguous Genitalia," *Comprehensive Therapy* 18, no. 1 (1992): 22-5.

21. A.E. Lang et al., "Posteroventral Medial Pallidotomy in Advanced Parkin-

son's Disease," *New England Journal of Medicine* 337, no. 15 (9 October 1997): 1036-42.

22. See, e.g., M.H. Freeston et al., "Cognitive-Behavioral Treatment of Obsessive Thoughts: A Controlled Study," *Journal of Consulting and Clinical Psychology* 65 (1997): 405.

23. J. Lock, "Treatment of Homophobia in a Gay Male Adolescent," *American Journal of Psychotherapy* 52, no. 2 (1998): 202-14.

24. J. Goodall, "Helping a Child to Understand Her Own Testicular Feminization, *Lancet* 337, no. 8732 (5 January 1991): 33-5. For a debate on whether—as opposed to how—these individuals should be told, see B.P.M. Inoque, R. Taraszewski, and S. Elias, "The Whole Truth and Nothing but the Truth," *Hastings Center Report* 18, no.5 (October/November 1988): 34-36.

25. "AIS causes XY fetuses to develop female external genitalia. Their testes produce androgens, but, because of a cellular abnormality that partially or completely inhibits response to the hormone, gestational development is unaffected and proceeds toward a female external morphology at birth." K. Kipnis and M. Diamond, "Pediatric Ethics and the Surgical Assignment of Sex," chapter 17 of this book.

26. Both of these interventions involve not only giving information, but presenting it in its most optimistic light. Some might consider this to be implicit deception. If it is deception, however, it may be justifiable because it is necessary to create the optimism to become a self-fulfilling prophecy.

Watson and Money support this same approach when counseling persons with Turner's Syndrome. Typically, these girls have no ovaries and are short in stature. These authors assert: "Avoid at all costs the presumption of making a prophecy! The counselor can disclose the probability of sterility and indicate that it is expected that the patient will achieve motherhood by adoption. Told in this way, the idea of parenthood remains intact. . . . This statement, in positive terms . . . can have the effect of self-fulfilling prophecy." M.A. Watson and J. Money, "Behavior Cytogenics and Turner's Syndrome: A New Principle in Counseling and Psychotherapy," *American Journal of Psychotherapy* 24 (1975): 166-78, at 171 and 176.

27. See, for example, V. DiBenedetto et al., "The Anterior Sagittal Transanorectal Approach: A Modified Approach to 1-Stage Clitoral Vaginoplasty in Severely Masculinized Female Pseudohermaphrodites: Preliminary Results," *Journal of Urology* 157 (January 1997): 330-32; and E.M.F. Costa et al., "Management of Ambiguous Genitalia in Pseudohermaphrodites: New Perspectives on Vaginal Dilation," *Fertility and Sterility* 67, no. 2 (February 1997): 229-32.

28. Chase, "Surgical Progress," see note 4 above.

29. For example, in regard to women: B.R. Komisaruk, C.A. Gerdes, and B. Whipple, " 'Complete' Spinal Cord Injury Does Not Block Perceptual Responses to Genital Self-Stimulation in Women," *Archives of Neurology* 54 (December 1997): 1513-20.

In regard to men: "there is a widely held belief that no level of sexual response below complete tumescence is fully useful, adequate, or satisfying . . . the SCI men had much the same feelings of arousal as the non-SCI men. Such a finding challenges claims that . . . feelings of sexual arousal . . . are lessened by spinal cord injury." S. Kennedy and R. Over, "Psychophysiological Assessment of Male Sexual Arousal Following Spinal Cord Injury," *Archives of Sexual Behavior* 19, no. 1 (1990): 15-26, at 24 and 25.

30. M.L. Sipski, C.J. Alexander, and R.C. Rosen, "Orgasm in Women with Spinal Cord Injuries: Laboratory-Based Assessment," *Archives of Physical and Medical Rehabilitation* 76 (1995): 1097-102. "This information should help to dispel the myth that women with SCI, especially those with complete injuries, cannot achieve orgasm." Ibid., 1101.

31. "There are numerous subjective reports of women who have erotogenic areas in places where previously stimulation of these areas produced little or no excitement." B. Whipple, C.A. Gerdes, and B.R. Komisaruk, "Sexual Response to Self-stimulation in Women with Complete Spinal Cord Injury," *Journal of Sex Research* 33, no. 3 (1996): 231-40, at 232.

32. "The rapid occurrence of such precise, functionally effective sprouting has never been documented in the adult human brain and it produces some grounds for optimism." V.S. Ramachandran, "Behavioral and Magneto-encephalographic Correlates of Plasticity in the Adult Human Brain," *Proceedings of the National Academy of Sciences, USA* 90 (1993): 10413-20, at 10420. Of course, surgery in early infancy may prevent women from acquiring the capacity to have orgasms later in life, because the trophic influences necessary for critical brain parts may not develop.

33. A cultural example is offered by the Navaho. Intersexual persons are "made heads of the family and are given control of family property, because " 'They know everything.'" C. Elliott, "Why Can't We Go on as Three?" *Hastings Center Report* 28, no. 3 (May-June 1998): 36-39, at 37.

34. *You Don't Know Dick* (Montreal, P.Q., Canada: Films Transit) videotape. The address for Films Transit is 402 E. Notre Dame, Montreal, P.Q., H2Y 1C8, Canada. The film was shown at the American Psychiatric Association Annual Meeting in May 1998 in Toronto, Ont., Canada.

35. "It is intriguing in regard to this possibility that in a study involving women with spinal cord injuries (SCI), *the SCI subjects acknowledged a better balance of masculine and feminine characteristics than did the able-bodied women. This balance tends to be associated with more healthy sexual relationships*" [italic added]. Sipski, Alexander, and Rosen, "Orgasm in Women," see note 30 above, p. 1101.

36. This account is from J. Colapinto, "The Truth about John/Joan," *Rolling Stone* (11 December 1997): 56-97.

Contributors

TAMARA ALEXANDER has been wedded in spirit to Max Beck for more than five years. The couple make their home in Atlanta, Georgia, where they are renovating their historic home, surviving the antics of their three cats, and planning for a baby.

D. CAMERON is a former teacher and social worker. His current interests are historical renovation; individual creative expression through arts, crafts, and clowning; and gardening. He has been a mainstay volunteer in the ISNA San Francisco office since 1996.

CHERYL CHASE is Executive Director of the Intersex Society of North America, which can be contacted at info@isna.org or via its website, <http://www.isna.org>.

MARTHA COVENTRY writes about family and place, nature and love; her work appears in the national press and various anthologies. A memoir that explores her clitoridectomy and its aftermath will be published in 2000. She lives in Minneapolis, Minnesota, with her two daughters.

ROBERT A. CROUCH, MA, is a Doctoral Student in the Cocoran Department of Philosophy at the University of Virginia in Charlottesville. His research interests are in bioethics, political and moral philosophy, and the philosophy of science.

HOWARD DEVORE, PhD, is a Clinical Psychologist and Certified Sex Therapist in the San Francisco Bay Area, and has worked with ISNA since its inception. He has been out as an intersexed person since 1984, and works for change in the standard of care for the treatment of intersex infants.

MILTON DIAMOND, PhD, is a Professor in the Department of Anatomy and Reproductive Biology at the John A. Burns School of Medicine at the University of Hawaii in Manoa, and is Director of the Pacific Center for Sex and Society.

ALICE DOMURAT DREGER, PhD, is an Assistant Professor of Science and Technology Studies in the Lyman Briggs School, and is Adjunct Faculty in the Center for Ethics and Humanities in the Life Sciences at Michigan State University in East Lansing.

SHERRI A. GROVEMAN is the U.S. Representative of the AIS Support Group, which can be contacted at aissg@aol.com or via its website at < http://www.medhelp.org/www/ais >.

HALE HAWBECKER is a Washington, D.C., attorney who works for the Environmental Protection Agency Office of General Counsel. He received the 1999 EPA Employee Recognition Award for outstanding community service for the work he has done with intersexed people.

HELENA HARMON-SMITH is the Founder of the Hermaphrodite Education and Listening Post (HELP) in Jacksonville, Florida. She is the mother of an intersexed child.

EDMUND G. HOWE, MD, JD, is a Professor of Psychiatry and the Director of Programs in Medical Ethics at the Uniformed Services University of the Health Sciences in Bethesda, Maryland; he is Editor in Chief of *The Journal of Clinical Ethics.*

KIM lives in the Midwest with her partner and daughter, with whom she shares artistic talents and interests. She is currently working on an art project about gender, which she hopes will educate people about intersex issues.

KENNETH KIPNIS, PhD, is a Professor in the Department of Philosophy at the University of Hawaii in Manoa.

ANGELA MORENO is an intersex activist with the eerie coincidence of a day job in the Surgery Department of a hospital in Peoria, Illinois, and is busy establishing an Illinois chapter of the Intersex Society. She enjoys volunteering for a lesbian/gay youth organization and feeding her friends.

SVEN NICHOLSON lives amidst California valley oaks, providing translation services from his home to clients worldwide via the internet, as he listens to squirrels and jays and a pair of red-shouldered hawks.

SHARON E. PREVES, PhD, is an Assistant Professor of Sociology at Grand Valley State University in Allendale, Michigan.

WILLIAM G. REINER, MD, is an Assistant Professor of Child and Adolescent Psychiatry at Johns Hopkins University in Baltimore, Maryland.

JUSTINE MARUT SCHOBER, MD, is a Pediatric Urologist at Hamot Medical Center in Erie, Pennsylvania.

KIIRA TRIEA has expressed herself personally and politically as an intersex activist since 1993; current work includes educational speaking, a paper relating medical methodologies to actual outcomes of adult intersexuals, and co-producing and co-directing a documentary on intersexuality.

HEIDI WALCUTT, who lives in the American West, has been helping to change the treatment of intersex since 1995. She is working on finding naturopathic and holistic cures to daily ailments, increasing her spirituality, fulfilling her life contract, and learning to enjoy life with her lover.

BRUCE E. WILSON, MD, is a Pediatric Endocrinologist at DeVos Children's Hospital in Grand Rapids, Michigan, and is an Associate Professor in the Department of Pediatrics and Human Development at Michigan State University in East Lansing.

Photograph Credits

Page 4—Alice Domurat Dreger and Aron Sousa by Gustine Farmer, used with permission.

Pages 7 and 8—Figures 1-1 and 1-2 originally appeared in T. Tuffier and A. Lapointe, "L'Hermaphrodisme: Ses variétés et ses conséquences pour la pratique médicale (d'après un cas personnel)," *Revue de gynécologie et de chirurgie abdominale* 17 (1911): 209-68. Prints courtesy of the Wangensteen Historical Library at the University of Minnesota, Minneapolis.

Page 50—Sharon E. Preves by Nico Taranovsky, used with permission.

Page 70—Martha Coventry, used with permission.

Page 78—Howard Devore by Steven Underhill, used with permission.

Page 90—D. Cameron, before testosterone treatment, by Steve Timlin, used with permission.

Page 92—D. Cameron, after testosterone treatment, by Peter Tannen, used with permission.

Page 98—Kim, used with permission.

Page 102—Tamara Alexander and Max Beck by Tanya Alexander, used with permission.

Page 110—Hale Hawbecker, used with permission.

Page 140—Kiira Triea by Shelley Primrose, used with permission.

Page 146—Cheryl Chase by Asako Sugai, used with permission.

Page 156—(A) is reprinted from K. Newman, J. Randolph, and K. Anderson, "The Surgical Management of Infants and Children with Ambiguous Genitalia: Lessons Learned from 25 Years," *Annals of Surgery* 215, no. 6 (1992): 644-53, at 647, fig. 6, © 1992 by Lippincott Williams & Wilkins, used with permission; (B), (C), and (D) © 1998 by ISNA, used with permission.

Page 172—Kenneth Kipnis by Starr Holley, used with permission.

Page 174—Milton Diamond by Sara Diamond, used with permission.

Page 210—Edmund G. Howe and Chelsea Howe, by Joyce St. Giermaine, used with permission.